DISEASE AND DIAGNOSIS FOR THE ACUPUNCTURIST

An advanced guide for practitioners of acupuncture which explains the diagnostic techniques to be employed in the practice of acupuncture for those using traditional methods.

DISEASE AND DIAGNOSIS FOR THE ACUPUNCTURIST

An Advanced Guide to Traditional Diagnostic Techniques

by

Graham Player
Dip. Ac.

THORSONS PUBLISHERS LIMITED
Wellingborough, Northamptonshire

THORSONS PUBLISHERS INC.
New York

First published 1984

© GRAHAM PLAYER 1984

British Library Cataloguing in Publication Data

Player, Graham
    Disease and diagnosis for the acupuncturist.
    1. Acupuncture
    I. Title
    615.8'92   RM184

    ISBN 0-7225-0822-0

Thorsons Publishers Inc. are distributed to the trade by Inner Traditions International Ltd., 377 Park Avenue South, New York, NY 10016.

Printed and bound in Great Britain

CONTENTS

		Page
Introduction		7
1.	UNDERSTANDING DISEASE	9
2.	SOME BASIC PHYSIOLOGY	11
	2.1 Yin and Yang Functions of the Organs	11
	2.2 Fluid, Chi and Blood	12
	2.3 Chi and Yang	17
	2.4 Blood and Yin	17
3.	DIFFERENTIATION OF DISEASE	19
	3.1 Cold Illness	20
	3.2 Hot Illness	20
	3.3 Empty Illness	23
	3.4 Full Illness	23
	3.5 External Illness	25
	3.6 Internal Illness	26
	3.7 Yin Illness	28
	3.8 Yang Illness	28
	3.9 The Six Excesses	28
4.	DIAGNOSIS	32
	4.1 Occupation	32
	4.2 Major Complaints	32
	4.3 History of Onset	33
	4.4 Past History	33
	4.5 Shen	33
	4.6 Posture or Physical Condition	34
	4.7 Facial Observation	34

4.8   Eyes   36
4.9   Nose   37
4.10 Mouth   37
4.11 Lips   38
4.12 Teeth and Gums   38
4.13 Skin   39
4.14 Throat   39
4.15 Nails   39
4.16 Ears   40
4.17 Drinking and Thirst   40
4.18 Diet   40
4.19 Sleeping Pattern   41
4.20 Urine   42
4.21 Faeces   42
4.22 Sputum and Nasal Mucus   43
4.23 Menstruation   43
4.24 Tongue Condition   43
4.25 Pulse Diagnosis   52
4.26 General Body Signs   54

5. Physiology of Points   57

6. Indication Reference   116

    Bibliography   143

    General Index   144

INTRODUCTION

This book is based on the traditional Chinese theories of medicine and has been written primarily as a useful guide to diagnostic techniques to be employed in the practice of acupuncture for those practicing the traditional methods.

As such, it is not recommended for the layman or the new student of acupuncture, but more for the practitioner or near graduate. However the student may derive some benefit from the 'Point Physiology' section.

I have not attempted any explanation of the following topics which can be read from a number of books currently available, and I consider a knowledge of these topics to be an essential prerequisite or corequisite to this book in order to fully benefit from its content:

> Acupuncture Theory
> Point Location
> The Meridians — Main Meridians
> Luo Meridians
> 8 Extra Meridians
> Muscle Meridians
> Divergent Meridians
> The Five Elements - Their Cycles, Foods and Influences on the Body
> Chi Production
> Command, Antique, Window of the Sky, Hung, Sea, Influential, Meeting and Alarm Points
> The Six Divisions and the Progression of Disease
> The Pulses
> Needle, Moxa and Electro Acupuncture Techniques
> Basic Anatomy and Physiology

Instead, I have based this book on the diagnostic techniques, a subject which I feel cannot be over emphasized in the study of acupuncture or any other mode of Chinese medicine. This is particularly true for the student who is unfamiliar with Western medicine and therefore unfamiliar with disease and diagnosis in any form. A knowledge of acupuncture treatment is useless without the knowledge to diagnose the problem.

At the end of the book I have included a section called 'Point Physiology' which is a compendium of acupuncture points in alphabetic sequence, showing for each point a list of important information to consider when selecting the appropriate point. (This information does not include the basic command point details which is assumed knowledge).

Following this is an 'Indication Reference' section which represents the 'indication' category from the Point Physiology section, but this time in indication sequence rather than point sequence. This section when used in conjunction with the Point Physiology section is designed to initiate some thought as to why a particular point may be beneficial to select. It is definitely not designed to present a formula for treatment in symptomatic acupuncture.

It seems to me that a lot of Western practitioners of acupuncture use mostly 'symptomatic' acupuncture which definitely is an important facet of acupuncture, however I feel it should not form the basis of treatment but rather a technique to 'fall back' on in those instances when no other treatment can be devised from the wholistic approach. This predominately symptomatic approach may be due to a lack of understanding of adequate diagnostic techniques.

I do not advocate that acupuncture is a panacea for all ailments but rather an integral adjunct for maintaining health in a lot of cases, together with many other modes of treatment, in which I include such things as:

> Diet
> Exercise
> Balanced emotional states and living standards
> Western medicine
> Education
> and many 'alternative' therapies

I feel that in a lot of cases, acupuncture alone without the introduction of other considerations such as the above may have little effect.

I hope that this book makes at least a small contribution toward the dissemination of knowledge in the field of acupuncture and Chinese medicine.

1. UNDERSTANDING DISEASE

Chinese traditional medicine was influenced by the belief that man is a microcosm of the universe influenced by Tao, a principle operating through the two opposing forces yin and yang.

In the universe the harmonious working of the two forces of yin and yang expressed itself in the rising and setting of the sun, the growing and ripening of crops, and in all natural phenomena. An imbalance of yin and yang led to droughts, floods and other natural disasters.

Similarly within man, it is believed that health depends on the harmonious balance of yin and yang. This belief in the yin/yang harmony is further carried through to the functions within the body. That is, each yin function is believed to have a balancing yang function in order to maintain balance and harmony. For example:

Yin Function	Balancing Yang Function
Stomach makes energy go down.	Spleen makes energy go up.
Kidney stores energy.	Liver disperses.
Kidney grabs the energy.	Lung makes energy go down and circulate.

Heart co-ordinates all these activities

The cause of this yin/yang imbalance can be as a result of any of the following factors:

(a) mental and emotional activity,

   (b) natural climatic factors - heat, dampness, dryness, cold, wind,

   (c) biological factors - pathogenic virus, bacteria, fungi, tapeworm, etc.,

   (d) chemical factors - acids, alkalis, pharmaceuticals, toxins,

   (e) physical factors - injuries, excess work,

   (f) hereditary factors,

   (g) diet and bad eating habits.

This causative factor or influence comes into conflict eventually with the primary chi of the body (ying or nourishing chi) and may result in any of the following:

   (a) Ying chi overcomes the influence either because the influence is too weak or the ying is very strong. This could produce acute symptoms while the body is combatting the evil influence but the disease eventually subsides.

   (b) Evil influence overcomes the ying chi due to the ying being weak. This could result in death if the influence is strong enough.

   (c) Neither the influence or the ying chi is overcome and the conflict continues over a long period resulting in a chronic disease.

2. SOME BASIC PHYSIOLOGY

2.1 Yin and Yang Functions of the Organs

Traditional Chinese medicine teaches the belief that each organ has an effect on and interacts with body tissues, sense organs, seasons, etc., as learnt from the 'concordances'. It is most important that the practitioner has a thorough knowledge of these concordances, which form the basis of diagnosis.

It is also of great importance that the functioning of each organ be understood in relation to its yin function and yang function. This can quite simply be deduced given the overall function of the organ, and the following table briefly presents some differentiation of the tsang organs:

Organ	Yin Function	Yang Function
Heart	Controls organ activities.	Moves the blood.
Spleen	Governs the blood and keeps it in the vessels.	Transformation and transportation. Moves energy up to the lungs.
Lung	Drives chen chi down to circulate in the body. Sends fluids down from the spleen to the kidney.	Separates the good of the air from the bad (oxygen and carbon dioxide). Makes chen chi from ku chi and cosmic chi. Brings energy to the outside of the body (controls wei chi).

Organ	Yin Function	Yang Function
Yin Kidney (Fluid)	Receives the pure fluids (some of which has been sent from the lungs).	Divides and transforms the fluid into pure — which eventually circulates with wei chi moisturizing the skin and flesh; and also circulates with ying chi forming the internal lubricants of tendons, joints, spinal and brain fluid. Impure — which forms the body fluids (sweat, saliva, mucus, urine, tears). Evaporates some fluid back up to moisten the lungs.
Yang Kidney (Energy)	Stores surplus chen chi as ching chi. Stores surplus ching chi as tsing (sexual) chi.	Produces tsing (sexual) chi. Transforms impure chi from the colon and small intestine into wei chi.
Liver	Stores blood. Keeps blood in the head.	Releases blood. Moistens the eyes, tendons and muscles.

2.2 Fluid, Chi and Blood

The amount of **fluid** in the body depends mainly on the amount of food and water digested. The liquid in the stomach is metabolized by the action of the yin fluid already there. Too much or not enough fluid in the body upsets the yin/yang balance in the system.

Any failure in this system of fluid control and circulation can lead to illness and it is said that diabetes and edema are both conditions of the fluid.

The seasons also influence the amount of fluid in the body as perspiration increases in the summer and urination increases in the winter.

Chi is one of the fundamental concepts of Chinese medicine. It represents a system of forces in the body which

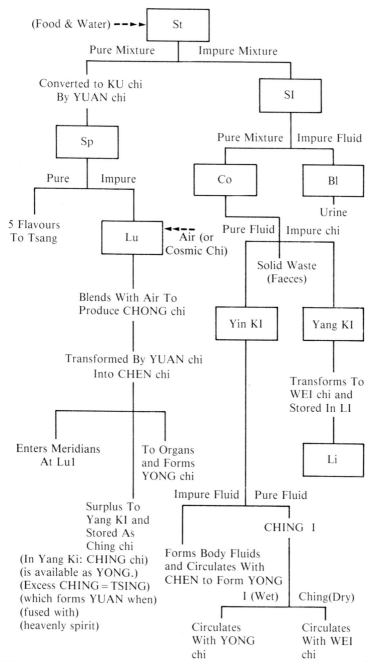

Chi Production and Circulation

enable man to move, breathe, think, digest food, etc. The interaction of these forces regulates all the functions of the body.

Chi is created by breathing and eating. The chi inhaled with the air is extracted by the lungs, and the chi in food and water is extracted by the stomach and spleen.

Chi causes the blood to circulate and the fluid to be disseminated throughout the body and excreted as urine and sweat. It transforms the food we eat into more chi, blood fluid etc., and the organs of the body are active only because of the energy of chi. It activates the process of digestion and regulates the capacity of the intestines to absorb only those substances which the body needs and to excrete the remainder.

(Refer to the preceding diagram on chi, its production and circulation.)

Blood is formed from the combination of ching I and ying chi in the middle warmer (spleen and stomach). Chi controls the movement of blood - if chi moves then the blood moves. It is said that in addition to ying chi, blood also circulates in the meridians - the ying chi representing the yang element and the blood representing the yin element. Each meridian has a certain proportion of chi and blood, as is known from the six divisions.

Some symptoms of chi and blood disorders are as follows:

Empty Chi
Can produce tiredness, pale face and empty pulse. The organs usually affected by empty chi, and their associated symptoms are:

Heart   — palpitations
                intermittent or knotted pulse

Spleen — weak limbs
             pale yellow face
             watery stools
             diminished appetite
             food improperly transformed

Lung — shallow respiration
empty cough
untalkative
empty pulse

Kidney — tinnitus
dizziness
libido diminished
incontinence or inability to complete
urination

Stagnant Chi
Chi should always circulate, but it may be stuck in the
meridians by emotions (particularly grief), diet
(particularly greasy, cold foods), pathogens, causing
soreness and pain, or a feeling of fullness. Pain due to
stagnant chi is not constant, it is sometimes intense and
sometimes not. It tends to disperse on pressure and moves
around. It often becomes worse due to emotions. As a
general rule, pain and swelling usually indicate that
something is stagnant or stuck.

Stagnant Blood
Blood should always flow smoothly but it may be stuck or
stagnant due to:

chi being stagnant
empty chi
heat
cold
trauma

Symptoms of stagnant blood may be:

soreness pain and swelling (similar to stagnant chi, but
the differentiation is that it does not disperse on
pressure. The pain is more severe, the location more
fixed and is often accompanied by haemorrhage)
tendency to cyanosis
darkening complexion
pulse obstructed
tongue darkish purplish with red spots
(Note: Bleeding of points assists the yang function of
moving stagnant blood.)

Empty Blood
This may be due to such things as:

> middle heater not performing its transformation
>   function
> haemorrhaging
> stagnant blood

and could cause:

> insomnia
> dizziness (internal wind rising)
> spots in front of the eyes (due to no blood in the liver)
> tongue pale and maybe cold, with little or no moss
> thin pulse
> face ashen yellow or dull pale
> fingernails white
> legs and feet numb

It is possible to have empty yin without having empty blood. Empty blood will have more cold symptoms whereas empty yin will have more hot symptoms. Examine the tongue especially, in empty chi or blood there may be a tendency towards sluggish intestines, or mucus.

Hot Blood
This is usually due to an external cause but occasionally internal. Heat injures the meridians and causes the blood to spill (or rise) to the surface and may show symptoms of:

> rashes
> hives
> nose bleed
> skin problems
> irritability
> thirst
> scarlet red tongue
> pulse fast and possibly full

Because of the common origin of fluid, blood and chi it is important to appreciate that a deficiency of fluid, for example, will produce a corresponding deficiency of chi and blood, and vice versa.

2.3 Chi and Yang

Chi is part of the yang balance within the body and when an empty chi condition exists, this implies a slight increase in the yin level of the body and a decrease in the yang level. This is confirmed by looking back at the empty chi symptoms previously mentioned.   .

A larger decrease in the yang level (therefore a further increase in the yin level) is known as empty yang which is a more severe condition than empty chi and produces yin symptoms of :

> bright pale face
> low spirit
> daytime sweat
> chi empty
> fear of the cold
> four limbs cold
> face greyish and dark under the eyes
> pulse very slow and empty

A still further decrease in the yang level (implying a further increase in the yin level) is known as vanquished yang. This is an even more severe condition than empty yang and occurs classically in the case of shock, when the yang is said to flee, and can cause:

> oily sweat
> no thirst, but wants to sip warm water
> limbs cold and body feels cold
> respiration minute
> tongue is white and moist
> pulse very minute, without strength and sometimes
>   imperceptible

2.4 Blood and Yin

Blood is part of the yin balance within the body and blood may be associated with warmth, therefore when an empty blood condition exists there are more cold symptoms prevalent as is confirmed by looking back at the empty blood symptoms previously mentioned.

Empty yin is a condition where the yin level in the body is

depleted, which implies an excess yang level, and produces apparent yang symptoms of:

    dry mouth
    five hearts are hot
    night sweating
    tongue reddish
    pulse thin and fast

A further decrease in the yin level with a corresponding increase in the yang level produces a vanquished yin condition. This is a more serious condition than empty yin and maybe caused by great loss of body fluids or blood (both yin), or heat-stroke, and can cause:

    profuse sweating
    no strength in the body
    craves cold and dislikes heat
    skin burning hot
    dry tongue
    coarse respiration
    warm limbs
    red tongue with little moss, and dry
    pulse flooding (as yang is exploding out of the body),
        or thin and fast

3. DIFFERENTIATION OF DISEASE

Traditionally there are eight principles of discrimination or disease classification:

Li (Internal) Piao (External)	These classifications differentiate the site (internal or external) and the extent and seriousness of the disease.
Han (Cold) Je (Hot)	Cold and hot are used to differentiate the nature of the disease.
Hsu (Empty) Shih (Full)	These are indicators used to differentiate the extent or seriousness of the illness and the resistance of the human body. They are necessary to understand the type of treatment.
Yin Yang	These classify the illness. On the basis of clinical manifestations, the diagnosis of all diseases may be divided into two great categories - Yin and Yang.

These classifications of illnesses are necessary to be made in order to understand the direction of change of the disease and in order to treat at the proper site. The appropriate treatment depends on the correct differentiation and incorrect diagnosis may result in aggravation of the condition.

A more detailed description of the above mentioned eight principles follows and to gain a more thorough understanding of these principles, knowledge of the three diagnostic techniques below is imperative:

(a) tongue diagnosis

(b) pulse diagnosis

(c) techniques of visual observation of related parts of the patients body and its secretions, excretions, etc.

together with an understanding of the physiology of the human body according to traditional Chinese theory.

Sometimes it may be very difficult to distinguish and classify an illness from the symptoms presented by the patient, and it is important to note that observations in these cases should take precedence over the symptoms, especially observations of the pulse and tongue.

3.1 Cold Illness
This is usually caused by penetration of cold from outside and is characterized by:

diminished physiological function
decreased energy
decreased resistance to pathogens
pale tongue with white moist moss
slow pulse

Refer to the distinction of hot and cold symptoms below.

3.2 Hot Illness
This is due mostly to invasion of noxious heat from outside or overactive reaction of the human body. The principle symptoms being:

hyperactive physiological function
increased energy
over-reaction to pathogens
red tongue with yellow dry moss
fast pulse

Distinction Between Cold and Hot Symptoms
There are many other symptoms which help to distinguish between a hot and cold illness, some of which are:

Cold Symptom	Hot Symptom	Remarks
Usually dreads cold.	Dreads heat but occasionally may dread cold.	
Wears more clothes and likes more bed clothes.	Wears few clothes or few bed clothes.	Dread of cold and not using cooling agents in the height of summer is a cold symptom. Extending hands and feet out of the bed covers even in cool/cold weather is a hot symptom.
Not thirsty, but likes hot drinks.	Thirsty and craves cold drinks.	Cold illness can sometimes produce a thirst but only to sip not to swallow. In fact the body doesn't suffer from lack of saliva and fluid but rather a deficiency of yang and as a result saliva and fluid cannot be dispersed so thirst is relative, not actual. Some cases of hot illness may consume large quantities of hot rather than cold drinks. Care should be taken to rule out mere habitual preference. Thirst

Cold Symptom	Hot Symptom	Remarks
		following heavy perspiration or diarrhoea is a natural response to loss of body fluid and as such does not constitute a hot illness.
Urine is abundant and clear.	Small amount of yellow/red urine.	In summer or with small intake of water, urine is normally less, and less a deep yellow colour.
Diarrhoea.	Constipation.	Loose and thin stool with foul odour and yellow colour is a hot symptom. Loose thin stool containing undigested food, if acute, belongs to hot. Habitual constipation or constipation of the aged due to withered blood and damaged fluids should not be classed as hot. Pellets of mucus covering stool in the case of a spastic colon should not be considered a hot symptom.
Facial pallor.	Facial flushing.	Pallor is constant for a cold illness. Severe chill of a hot illness may also show pallor but this is transient

Cold Symptom	Hot Symptom	Remarks
		only. Because of fading vital energy in a cold illness, false (empty) yang floats up and produces transient facial flushing.
Coolness or coldness of limbs.	Warmness of limbs.	In a cold illness the extremities may warm slightly after hot food or drink.
White tongue with moist white moss.	Red tongue with dry or yellow moss.	Red tongue after hot food or drink is not a hot symptom and a moist tongue after constant drinking is not a cold symptom.
Slow pulse.	Fast pulse.	Pulse is not necessarily slow in a cold illness. In severe pain caused by cold the pulse may even be quickened.

3.3 Empty Illness

This is more a chronic illness where the vital chi has been exhausted resulting in a decrease of body function and a lowered resistance.

Refer to the distinction of empty and full symptoms below.

3.4 Full Illness

This is usually an acute illness of recent onset and short duration, and body functions, in normally healthy individuals, are overactive due to an excess of noxious chi.

Some typical causes of a full illness may be such things as:

accumulation of mucus
cold or greasy foods

accumulation of dampness
stagnant chi
stagnant blood

Distinction Between Empty and Full Symptoms

Empty Symptom	Full Symptom	Remarks
Withered face.	Flushed face.	Flushing, especially over the maxilla occurs in the afternoon in a yin empty illness - this is a false yang sign. Exercise, hot food, etc., can cause flushing.
Low spirit.	Good spirit.	A false spirit can show in the last stages of an empty illness and indicates that yang is escaping from the body (a critical sign).
Soft voice and apprehensive to talk.	Loud voice.	
Weak protrusion of tongue. Maybe no tongue moss. Weak pulse.	Forceful protrusion of tongue. Tongue moss. Strong pulse.	
Shallow and short respiration, and short exhalation.	Coarse and full respiration with prolonged exhalation.	Shallow and short respiration may occur in a full illness if there is an accumulation of fluid in the thoracic cavity. Coarse and full respiration in an

Empty Symptom	Full Symptom	Remarks
		empty illness indicates poor prognosis as with shallow and short respiration in a full illness. These show sudden changes internally.
Joint soreness is aching.	Joint soreness is more acute and grabbing.	
Paroxysmal abdominal distention.	Constant abdominal distention.	Abdominal distention in the afternoon or evening is an empty symptom. Acute abdominal distention throughout the day with relief after flatulence is a full symptom.

When an elderly person develops full symptoms the practitioner should be careful about dispersing the energy as elderly people need their energy.

3.5 External Illness

This is generally the beginning stages of exposure (chills) and may be classified as external cold or external hot. External illnesses are more external, affecting meridians, tendons, skin, etc., producing general symptoms of:

floating pulse
tongue moss more than normal
fever, aches, etc.

External Cold

Cold symptoms are predominant producing as well as the above:

pronounced aches and pains
tight pulse
white and moist tongue moss
no perspiration

External Hot
Sensation of heat is heavier (not necessarily higher temperature but a more subjective heat) and as well as the above general symptoms, produces:

aches and pains not as pronounced
fast pulse
yellow thick and dry tongue moss
red tongue body or tip

A cold wind usually attacks through the skin producing aches and shivering.

A hot wind usually attacks through the nose and throat producing a sore throat and affects more the stomach and lung.

3.6 Internal Illness
Before recovery from its external manifestations, the illness may develop inside the body. It can also be caused by the emotions, an inside evil, heredity or poor diet.

Internal illnesses may be commonly classified as follows with their related symptoms. A general symptom of all internal illnesses is a deep pulse.

Internal Hot and Full Illness
This is common when an outside evil progresses inwards as in the yang ming stage of disease producing symptoms of:

internal pains
abdominal pains
maybe vomiting
high fever
no fear of the cold
much thirst
irritable and restless spirit
maybe sweating

yellow and thick tongue moss
fast and full pulse

Internal Cold Illness

This is not very common but the symptoms are:

pale face
fear of the cold - likes heat
limbs cold or numb
no thirst - maybe a desire to drink warm liquids
urine clear and abundant
tongue pale and moist
pulse slow

Internal Empty Illness

This is generally the end result of a long term illness (e.g., pneumonia) and indicates great weakness. Symptoms are:

tiredness
insufficient chi
low voice
dizziness (as most kidney energy is used up)
poor appetite
low spirit
shortness of breath
spots in front of the eyes
pulse thin and empty - it could be weak and floating as
    the last energy reserves float out (false yang)
tongue pale and possibly swollen

Half Internal and Half External Illness

When the illness has left the confines of external illness but before it reaches the level of an internal illness it is half internal and half external producing symptoms of both the internal and external variety and:

vomiting
no appetite
bitterness in the mouth
alternating hot and cold feeling
dry throat
wiry pulse

Internal and External Together
This is a complex contradiction produced by two situations:

(a) outside evil in the outside of the body remains there and goes inside at the same time.

(b) internal disharmony exists (e.g., spleen yang empty) and an outside evil attacks at the same time.

3.7 Yin Illness
Most empty, cold and internal illnesses are yin illnesses.

3.8 Yang Illness
Most full, hot and external illnesses are yang illnesses.

3.9 The Six Excesses
Now that the eight principles of disease differentiation as mentioned above are understood, another important facet of disease classification is worth mentioning, and that is classification according to climatic factors.

The Chinese tend to use the meteorological terminology (wind, cold, heat, dampness, summer heat, dryness) to sometimes classify disease even further. These terms convey to the western person the idea, for example of wind blowing and entering the body causing disease. This is a valid deduction, but the Chinese may also refer to wind (or any other climatic condition) as something originating inside the body; a concept quite foreign to the western person.

The six meteorological terms mentioned above are known to the Chinese as the six excesses and some brief symptomatology of each follows:

Wind
Wind diseases have an upward effect on the body, because wind is light and tends to float upwards (headache is often a wind problem). Basically a yang problem.

Wind generally can cause:

moving pain
dizziness
spasms

convulsions
prickly crawly feeling on the skin

Wind can be generated as a result of other conditions, for example:

excess liver yang can generate wind

Wind is always an excess condition, even if it is caused by a deficiency, so in treatment it is necessary to sedate wind. If a wind is very violent, liver fire is said to rise.

Symptoms of external wind:

fear of the wind
fevers (as the body attempts to drive the wind out)
headache
floating pulse
a cold wind attacks through the skin and can cause
    aches around the neck and shoulders
a hot wind attacks via the nose and throat causing
    a sore throat and stuffy nose

Symptoms of internal wind:

tinnitus
spasms
headache
pulse weak and empty

Cold
If cold attacks there is a desire to be warm and fear of the cold. Elderly people may feel emptiness and cold in the belly and back areas.
Cold tends to produce:

Clear fluids (e.g., watery stools)
stagnation of chi and/or blood usually causing
    violent pains
contraction
stiffness

difficulty in moving (e.g., rheumatic problems)
fever without sweat
tendency to aching in the body and bones
slow pulse
pale tongue
white face

Internal cold may be caused due to weak yang energy in the body (therefore an excess of yin). If an internal cold condition exists then the patient is more susceptible to attack by external cold. (Refer also to information on the cold illness in section 3.1).

Heat Fire
If heat attacks it may produce symptoms of:

fevers (usually high)
heat in the entire body
fear of the heat
craving for cold
flushed face
tongue body red with yellow moss
pulse fast
red, hot, swollen, painful skin problems, (e.g., boils)
body excretions - thick and hot
      - more forceful than in cold condition
      - more smelly than in cold condition (as
       heat tends to cause things to rot)

Heat very easily damages the body fluids and will show this as a rough pulse. If heat penetrates the meridians it can drive the blood out (e.g., heat penetrating the lungs may produce nasal haemorrhage).
 Refer also to information on the hot illness in section 3.2.

Dampness
Dampness tends to produce symptoms of:

damp skin with a moist cloth appearance
edema

heaviness and tiredness in the body
watery discharges
thick greasy moss on the tongue
pulse slow, slippery

External dampness is usually environmentally related, for example, sweating and not changing the dampened clothes. Internal dampness damages the spleen yang giving:

digestion problems
watery faeces
little urination

Dampness is usually difficult to cure and the symptoms remain static.

Summer Heat
This is the damp heat of summer and is a yang hot evil. It easily wastes or damages the chi and injures the fluids of the body.
Refer also to the information on the hot illness in section 3.2.

Dryness
Dryness attacks the lungs producing:

dry nose
parched lips
nose bleed
dry cough without mucus
dry tongue and skin

Internal dryness may be due to empty yin in the body or insufficient body fluids due to sweating, vomiting, diarrhoea, etc.

4. DIAGNOSIS

In order to understand and recognize disease, the practitioner must thoroughly study his patients. By using such techniques as observation, listening, questioning and palpation, the practitioner can obtain significant data, on the basis of which he can apply the theories of disease differentiation and arrive at a correct diagnosis.

To obtain the relevant data about the patient, the practitioner should seek the following information and make the following observations before formulating a treatment:

4.1 Occupation
Determine the occupation and evaluate if it requires:

excesses of:	which may affect the organs of:
concentration	earth
worry	metal
fear	water
sitting	spleen
standing	kidney
walking	heart
use of the eyes	liver
lying down	lung

4.2 Major Complaints
Determine why the patient is seeking treatment and all the current ailments he is presenting.

Ascertain likes and dislikes in regard to climatic conditions, and season and time of day the problems are worse.

Basically this will take the form of the patient presenting a comprehensive report of his current state of disease.

It is imperative that the patient also indicates any current treatments or medications he is having.

4.3 History of Onset

This information should cover the whole course of the current diseases from the time the patient became ill to the time he presented himself for treatment, and may assist the practitioner using his knowledge of disease progression.

4.4 Past History

To learn about the patients general health and his past illnesses a complete history should be taken.

This should include such things as major illnesses, operations, presence of scars, drugs taken, chronic ailments, allergies, etc., and should as far as possible be a chronological presentation, which may prove helpful in treating the current disease. That is, the practitioner may be able to perceive the diseases as they have passed through the five element cycle.

4.5 Shen

The practitioner should make an observation of the shen (i.e., spirit, vitality, energy, etc.) of the patient. An excess or deficiency of chen chi and the severity of the diseases can be evaluated by the condition of the shen.

For example, consideration should be given to such things:

as:	which may indicate problems with:
restless, angry	wood
nervous, timid	water
tension	wood
low voice	metal
talks a lot or husky voice	fire
limp and exhausted	yin
extroverted	yin empty
sad	metal, water
can't concentrate	earth
no confidence	water
giggling	fire
laughing, smiling	fire
indecisive	wood

4.6 Posture or Physical Condition
The patients general physical condition and body stamina should be observed through his body movements (walking, sitting, lying down, standing up) and body build.

Such things as:	may indicate problems in:
shoulders hunched forward	metal
sloping backward stance	underactive gall bladder
prominent shoulder blades	lung
shoulders not level	gall bladder
obesity	water
damp hands	earth
cold, limp hands	water

4.7 Facial Observation
The most important observation to make about the patient's face is colouring.

Red Face
The colour red is associated with heat and a red face indicates a hot illness with excess fire. If the patient has a high temperature or hypertension it then indicates surface heat.

If the face is red and there are hot flushes with delirious speech it is a sign of surface heat. Red cheeks in the afternoon indicates an insufficiency of yin and an excess of fire.

A red face which looks as if cosmetics have been applied, with hot flushes and some white colour indicates an insufficient and exhausted condition.

Yellow Face
Yellow indicates a damp empty condition most likely of the spleen.

A yellow face and a yellow tinge to the white of the eye represents jaundice.

— yang jaundice is when the complexion and skin appear damp and the colour of orange peel (usually from damp heat in the spleen).

— yin jaundice is when the skin is a darker older dull yellow colour indicating damp cold.

A faint yellow tinge to the eyeballs and face (called empty yellow) is seen when there is a spleen weakness, weak digestive system or empty chi of the spleen and stomach. If this is accompanied with a fatty appearance in the face it indicates mucus or dampness. Yellow dry and withered complexion indicates excess fire in the stomach (a burning stomach).

White Face
A white complexion indicates that the lungs are insufficient in energy (empty chi), and cold.

A bright white (and usually swollen and puffy) face is mostly empty yang or chi and is typically seen after great loss of blood.

A dull white (and usually thin) face indicates empty blood. A pale thin face with red cheeks and lips indicates empty yin and an excess of fire. When the complexion is pale like bone it means the chi energy of the lung is at an end.

White spots and patches indicates parasites, and white at the front of the ears indicates parasites.

A pale complexion with dark patches on the forehead and face is normal in a pregnant woman or a woman on the Pill. Greyish greenish white indicates shock (i.e., vanquished yang).

Black Face
A black complexion indicates that the kidney is insufficient or cold, or stagnant blood. There may also be numbness.

Black represents water which is cold; excess cold causes poor circulation which in turn causes pain. Therefore a black colour means cold and pain.

If the black colour appears dry and burnt then the patient is hot.

When the black colour is associated with a thin person it indicates that yin fire is causing internal injury.

Green and black which are light and dull indicates an insufficiency of yang chi.

Black represents an excess of yin and an insufficiency of yang which is a severe case.

If the complexion is dull black but there is lustre and radiance from the bridge to the tip of the nose it means that the illness is not as severe. However if the nose from the bridge to the tip is dry, this is a severe illness and recovery is difficult.

Green Face
A green complexion indicates liver wind cold. If there is pain this indicates stagnant chi or blood due to poor circulation.

Green with a blackish tinge indicates a very painful and cold case.

Green with white indicates empty wind.

Green with red indicates fire in the liver. If both these colours are dull it means obstructed fire.

Green face and lips indicates an excess of yin.

Other observations to make from the patients face are the lines. There is much disagreement about the meaning of the facial lines (even between the Su Wen and the Ling Shu) and as such they are not as reliable a tool as the facial colouring.

4.8 Observation of the Eyes
The eyes as a general rule should be used to confirm a primary diagnosis.

Pain, swelling and redness of the eyes usually indicates a full yang fire condition.

Swelling indicates wind.

Itching indicates wind and fire.

Dryness can indicate poor liver function, insufficient kidney yin or damaged fluids.

Photophobia with swelling indicates a fire problem (usually liver).

Photophobia without swelling indicates weak liver yin due to weak kidney yin.

Blurred vision indicates damage to the blood or yin.

Double vision indicates a weakness of liver and kidney energy.

If a child sleeps with its eyes slightly open this indicates a predisposition to wind problems (like convulsions due to lack of blood in the liver).

If an adult sleeps with eyes slightly open it indicates a spleen weakness which is not making enough blood for the liver to store (usually a chronic condition).

4.9 Observation of the Nose
Dry nostrils indicate heat or a wind condition of the lungs or a dry outside evil attacking the body. A red nose indicates wind heat of the spleen or lungs. A white nose indicates empty chi or a large blood loss. A black nose indicates involvement with the kidney. If only slightly black it indicates edema (spleen and kidney yang problem). Black and cold indicates a great amount of cold energy in the body.

A shining cold nose with oily skin is from poor digestion of the spleen (left over food in the body).

A swollen nose is a severe problem and is typically seen in alcoholics.

If the inside of the nose is painful it indicates fire in the lungs. An itchy nose indicates wind fire or parasites. Epistaxis (nose bleed) indicates liver or stomach fire attacking the lung.

4.10 Mouth
Loss of taste indicates a yin disease (energy of spleen insufficient).

A sweet taste indicates heat and dampness in the spleen. A bitter taste indicates fire in the heart or liver.

A sour taste is from poor digestion.

A sweet smelling breath is seen in the first stages of diabetes (stomach problem).

A foul smelling breath indicates fire in the stomach.

Much mucus in the mouth is caused by a weak spleen. Dryness in the mouth indicates yin energy very weak giving rise to stomach fire.

A sticky feeling in the mouth indicates dampness in the body.

A salty taste in the mouth indicates heat in the kidneys.

Drooling of saliva indicates an empty spleen, or stomach heat.

4.11 Lips
Whiteness of the lips is a lung condition or empty blood. Blackness of the lips is a kidney disease with extreme cold. Extreme redness indicates heart fire. If very red and dull it indicates problems with the circulatory aspects of the heart. Cyanozed lips indicate extreme cold or a very serious liver problem.

Dry lips indicate spleen fire, or damage to the fluids.

Swollen lips indicates a spleen problem.

4.12 Teeth and Gums
If there is a tendency to blackness after cleaning it indicates fire in the kidneys.

If the upper teeth are constantly dry (lips sticking to the teeth) it indicates stomach fire. If the lower teeth are dry it indicates colon or small intestine fire.

If the teeth decay easily it indicates excess wind and heat.

A light gum colour indicates blood loss.

A red gum colour indicates fire.

Slightly blue gums indicate poisoning from heavy metals.

Swollen gums indicate fire in the digestive system.

Loose teeth indicate kidney fire.

If the gums bleed after tooth brushing it may indicate fire in the stomach.

4.13 Skin
Scaliness of the skin indicates poor meridian circulation.

Swelling of the skin can be due to wind, water, fire or obstruction of chi.

Dull and old looking skin indicates a deficiency of chi or blood.

If the skin is loose or easily damaged it indicates weak lungs. The skin becoming leathery and rough is a severe lung problem.

Patches of leathery and painful skin indicate stagnant blood underneath.

4.14 Throat
The throat has a connection with the lungs and stomach.

A normal throat is pale red and glistening with no pain or swelling.

A red swollen and painful throat indicates heat in the lungs or stomach.

Ulceration of the throat indicates severe heat.

A greyish whitish covering on the throat which can be scraped off without causing bleeding is a stomach problem. If the covering does not come off without bleeding, diptheria may be indicated.

A minor sore throat without outside evil symptoms indicates kidney fire (i.e., a kidney yin deficiency).

4.15 Nails
The nails are an extension of the tendons and controlled by the liver. The normal colour of the nails should be red with a good lustre.

If liver blood is full then the patient will have healthy strong nails.

Thin, soft, cracked or caved in nails indicates an insufficiency of energy or blood.

If nails tend to splay or turn up noticeably it indicates a predisposition to arthritis.

Thin longtitudinal lines on the nails indicate empty blood and a predisposition to nervousness.

More pronounced fluting on the nails indicates the beginning of arthritis.

Soft nails are often connected with emotional problems.

White nails indicate empty blood.

Purple nails indicate stagnant blood (often associated with pain).

Very red nails indicate fire.

When the surface of the nail is pressed it should go white, but on the release of pressure it should return to the normal red colour. If the red colour does not return immediately it indicates empty blood.

4.16 Ears
A normal ear should be thick and have lustre. This means that there is a surplus of pre-natal kidney yin and that the body has a good reserve of energy.

If the ear is thin and dry it indicates that the pre-natal kidney yin is insufficient.

White ears indicates cold.

Green or black ears indicate pain.

A dry and black helix indicates empty kidney yin.

Swollen ears indicate a surplus of perverse energy.

4.17 **Drinking and Thirst**
A severe thirst indicates heat in the yang ming.

No thirst indicates cold or dampness inside.

Thirsty but not wanting to drink indicates internal heat and dampness or improper fluid circulation.

4.18 **Diet and Eating Habits**
If during an illness, the appetite increases it means that the chi of the stomach and spleen is improving. But if the appetite decreases it indicates the chi is declining. If the patients

condition feels better after eating it is an empty condition. If worse after eating it is a full condition. No appetite indicates fullness due to improper digestion, or constipation.

A hungry feeling but not wanting to eat indicates fire caused by mucus.

If the patient eats a lot but is still hungry it indicates stomach fire (possibly diabetes).

A distended feeling after eating indicates poor circulation of chi.

If only one type of food is craved it indicates parasites.

4.19 Sleeping Pattern
Oversleeping may indicate empty or weak yang, or damp mucus in the body.

Dreaming a lot indicates deficient kidney or liver yin. It could also be pericardium is empty and allows the spirit to escape.

If heart blood or yin is empty and the shen is disturbed it usually results in light sleep patterns.

Easily awakened indicates a disorder of the heart or gall bladder chi, empty yin (especially of the heart), or fire in the heart.

Waking and not knowing whether they have slept or not indicates fire in the yang ming.

Waking late, especially in yang people, indicates excess chi.

Insomnia may be due to:

(a) heart blood empty and the spirit can't be calmed,

(b) too much thinking which influences the spleen directly and the heart indirectly,

(c) liver and kidney yin empty,

(d) empty chi.

Chronic insomnia may be empty heart blood, or heart fire.

Wakefulness and early awakening usually indicates an active heart fire, deficient gall bladder energy, or weak energy in the aged.

4.20 **Urine**

Polyuria and nocturia indicate empty kidney yang.

Oliguria to anuria indicates great loss of fluid and maybe due to dysentry, diarrhoea, vomiting, weak kidney chi, bladder chi weak.

Incontinence can indicate weak kidney chi. Inability to complete urination can also indicate weak kidney chi or weak spleen chi.

Passing less urine than normal indicates edema.

The colour of the urine is also an important guide in diagnosis. Remember that the first urination in the morning is not a reliable aid as it is always more concentrated.

Yellow and dark indicates heat.

A small amount of blood in the urine indicates that damp heat in the bladder has accumulated and knotted up or excess sexual activity.

Yellow and muddy indicates damp heat.

Reddish tinge from extreme concentration indicates excess fire in the blood.

Clear urine indicates a cold condition or insufficient kidney yang.

4.21 **Faeces**

Watery yellowish faeces with a bad smell indicates damp heat in the spleen, stomach and intestines.

Soft, frequent, small in quantity often with blood present and a tight feeling in the rectum with burning indicates damp heat in the colon.

Constipation indicates a hot condition.

Diarrhoea, or undigested food in the faeces both indicate a cold condition (possibly a spleen yang problem).

A dry stool indicates heat or insufficient fluids.

A foul smell generally indicates heat.

4.22 Sputum and Nasal Mucus

If sputum is white, clear, thin, loose and easy to bring up, it indicates a cold condition.

Yellow or white and thick sputum indicates heat.

A small quantity of sputum difficult to bring up indicates fire and dryness.

A large quantity of sputum easy to bring up, which is white indicates cold and dampness; if yellow it indicates heat and dampness.

If the nose is running with a clear discharge, or the nose is just stuffed up it indicates that the lung energy is not circulating properly (usually seen in the early stages of an external wind or cold disease).

If the mucus is thick and yellow but only for a short while, it indicates the end of the disease as the body's energy is fighting back. If it remains thick and yellow it indicates a wind or heat attack.

4.23 Menstruation

If the period is often early, it indicates the blood has heat.

If often late, it may be cold in the blood or stagnant blood.

If it fluctuates it can indicate spleen empty, stagnant blood (accompanied by blood clotting and severe pain) or stagnant chi (accompanied by less severe pain).

Excessive bleeding indicates heat in the blood or empty chi (liver chi).

Scanty light bleeding indicates empty or stagnant blood.

Blood clots indicate chi or blood are stagnant.

4.24 Tongue Condition

Visual examination of the tongue is a useful diagnostic aid and is shown to be a reliable indicator, and confirms other diagnostic signs. It is not very prone to false symptoms and can be a good early warning indicator of impending disease as the tongue tends to show signs one step ahead of the disease.

By observing changes in the tongue the practitioner can observe the disease progression.

It is important to remember that food and temperature will change the colour of the tongue body, as will cigarettes, medicines, liquorice, etc. This should be taken into account when diagnosing. There are also some localized diseases where the tongue does not alter.

When observing the tongue the practitioner should consider its general characteristics, body colour and coating as follows:

General Characteristics
The normal tongue should be lively looking, soft and easy to articulate with. However if there is an illness there may be various changes to the tongue's characteristics, being:

(A) Oversized or Swollen Tongue
This is characterized by teeth marks on the tongue from being swollen and pressing against the teeth, and usually indicates an empty condition.

If the tongue is pale white and moist it indicates an empty cold condition and weak spleen and kidney yang.

Fresh red indicates heat in the heart or stomach and could include the pericardium.

Purple indicates heat or alcoholism.

Dark purple, almost bruised looking indicates stagnant blood.

Normal colour either indicates empty yang or damp heat in the spleen or stomach.

(B) Thin Tongue
If pale white then yin and yang, chi and blood are empty. If scarlet purple then yin is empty leading to empty fire. An old red colour indicates empty yin where blood and yin have dried up. This is usually seen in older women.

(C) Contracted Tongue
This tongue is characterized as being too short to get out of the mouth.

If a pale white colour it indicates cold contracting the tendons and muscles (liver chi deficient) or spleen and kidney both weak causing empty blood and chi (empty blood results in improper nourishment of the body, and empty chi results in nothing moving).

Deep red indicates heat has injured the fluids causing wind which inhibits the tongue coming out.

A contracted tongue may also be the result of heat from mucus preventing normal movement.

(D) Stiff Hard Tongue (like wood)
This may be caused by internal wind or full heat in the pericardium meridian.

If the tongue is very dry it indicates heat has injured the fluids.

(E) Soft Atrophy Type of Tongue
If pale it indicates heart and spleen chi and blood are empty.

If red and dry it indicates extreme heat has injured the fluids.

(F) Protruding Tongue
If pale it indicates empty chi or blood.

If not pale it indicates a full hot condition.

If the tongue always protrudes and touches the lips then the spleen is dry.

If the protruded tongue rests more to one side it indicates wind involvement.

(G) Numb Tongue
This can be due to yin empty giving rise to wind. If there is heat the tongue will be red.

If quite red it indicates an excess of the liver causing wind.

(H) Quivering or Trembling Tongue
This type of tongue is quite common and can indicate a deficiency situation (lack of chi).

If pale white then chi and blood are insufficient (maybe a vitamin or mineral deficiency).

If dark red or scarlet it indicates liver wind or extreme heat causing wind.

(I) **Cracked Tongue**

This is usually found in acute cases of disease.
If dry it indicates damaged body fluids.

If the colour is light and it is soft it is a mild case of insufficient kidney yin.

If the centre of the tongue is cracked, bleeding and ruptured it indicates empty blood.

TONGUE SHOWING AREAS CONTROLLED BY PARTICULAR ORGANS

(Back or Root of Tongue)

Kidney
Area

Li
&
GB

Spleen
&
Stomach
Area

Li
&
GB

Lu

Ht

(Tip of Tongue)

This organ reflected on the tongue surface is a reference only, for symptoms and should not be considered definite.

The tongue is the Spirit of the Heart and is related to the spleen. The heart, kidney, liver and spleen meridians go to the tongue and there are conflicting opinions as to which organs are reflected on the tongue body. One opinion is according to this diagram.

Colour of Tongue Body
The normal colour is slightly pale to redish, bright and moist looking.
However, in illness the colour may vary as follows:

(A) **Pale White**
   This generally indicates an empty cold condition with insufficient yang chi to push the blood up.

   If moist (maybe fluid dripping off or puddles of fluid) it indicates spleen yang weak. Therefore earth is not controlling water.

   If dry (i.e., less than the normal amount of moisture) it can indicate that spleen yang is deficient and not producing fluids leaving the body generally run down (kidney is likely to be involved).

   If mirrored finish it indicates empty blood for a long duration. This mirrored appearance usually begins in the middle of the tongue (spleen area) and progresses outwards.

(B) **Scarlet or Dark Red**
   This indicates heat in the body which has pushed too much blood into the tongue. The deeper the redness the more heat is indicated.

   If moist and a fresh red colour it indicates empty yin with yang floating up (i.e., false heat). If moist and an older red it indicates solid heat (the liver is the only organ that produces solid heat) and is often seen in alcoholics.

   If dry it indicates full heat.

   If mirrored appearance, it indicates yin and fluids have been seriously damaged. The main causes of this are incorrect treatment causing sweating, or purgatives used too frequently. It may also be the result of a long term illness where kidney yin has been wasted.

If red pimples, it indicates heat attacking the blood or secondarily, stagnant blood. The location of the pimples will be organ specific.

If white pimples raised from the tongue (convex) it indicates heat poison in the body (a very hot condition). Concave white pimples indicate empty spleen chi.

If purple to red blotches or spots which aren't raised it indicates severe heat is causing the blood and chi to be stagnant.

If there are thorns (sharp looking pimples) usually on the tip of the tongue, but perhaps the entire tongue, it indicates the upper warmer has excess heat.

(C) **Purple**

If scarlet to purple it indicates very deep severe heat damaging the fluids, characterized by a dry tongue. It may also be stagnant blood due to weak chi not moving the blood.

If greeny purply blue colour it indicates deep cold stagnating circulation of the blood or injury to internal organs.

If dark purple, almost grey and lacking brightness it may be:

> — a very severe heat inside causing fluids and blood to be dry and stagnant (tongue will be dry),

> — patient had a previous condition of stagnant blood (in this case tongue will not be too dry),

> — an alcoholic with a damp heat condition (moss will be greasy).

If bruised and cyanosed appearance it indicates stuck blood.

This is usually associated with extreme pain.

Tongue Coating or Moss
During digestion the digestive system vaporizes a small amount of dirty food that is not digested and this dirty chi is taken up with the spleen yang chi and forms moss on the tongue.

The quantity of moss can indicate the strength of the normal chi or how much evil chi is present.

Little or no moss indicates either the normal chi is empty and weak or there is no outside evil going in, or the patient hasn't eaten in the last twenty-four hours. As a rule of thumb, the thicker the moss the more the evil. Therefore chi problems are reflected in the tongue moss whereas blood problems are observed from other tongue characteristics.

Normal moss is thin and even, and covers the tongue or just the centre. Usually the moss in the middle or root of the tongue is just slightly thicker. It should appear to be rooted to the tongue and growing like grass.

If the moss appears not to be rooted to the tongue it indicates a more severe emptiness is present.

If the moss is in patches or pieces it indicates lack of harmony between the spleen and stomach.

If the moss is moist it indicates cold in the body from an external evil (dampness) or deficient spleen and kidney yang.

If the moss is dry it indicates an outside hot evil is beginning to injure the fluids. An extreme case of this will cause cracked moss as there is insufficient moisture to hold it together.

Greasy moss, seen mostly in the centre or root of the tongue indicates mucus.

Moss Colour
Normally the moss is thin, white and not too moist or dry. However, in a diseased state it may be reflected as follows:

(A) White
   If thin and moist it indicates excess water internally or a cold, damp external evil.

   If thin and dry it indicates an outside dry evil or empty yin.

If slightly thick it indicates internal cold damp or an external disease probably in Shao Yang.

If thick and greasy and not too wet or dry it can be:

— stuck food in the stomach or intestines,

— dirty or mucus dampness,

— a disorder of spleen yang.

If the patient also feels that the mouth is sticky and greasy it can indicate damp heat.

If thick and greasy and moist it indicates cold dampness or mucus present obstructing the fluid circulation.

If thick, greasy and dry it may indicate:

— stomach dry with damaged fluids, and mucus in the body,

— stomach chi weak causing stuckness of fluid, chi and food. Therefore the spleen won't be moving and there will be symptoms of accumulations,

— dampness has accumulated in the centre of the body and the yang is not strong enough to move it,

— heat internally even though history indicates an original cold disease.

If rough like sand, usually with cracks it indicates sudden internal heat.

If sticky, thick, greasy and pasty (like the coating of yogurt) it indicates dampness and mucus internally, usually accompanied by cold. If accompanied with a sweet taste and thick saliva it can be a cold disease that has turned into heat.

If snow-flaked it indicates extreme emptiness of spleen yang, and a poor prognosis.

If dirty looking with a greyish tinge it indicates stomach and kidney have empty yin leading to empty fire. If the body of the tongue is pale it could be stuck mucus and damp cold.

If one side normal and one side thick it may indicate a disease of Shao Yang, excess chi in the liver, or mucus on the sides of the chest.

If split back and front and heavy at the back it indicates the kidneys are not obstructed but a long standing mucus obstruction of the middle heater, or mucus or damp heat in the intestines. If heavy at the front it indicates weak stomach, spleen and kidneys.

(B) Yellow

Yellow indicates internal heat as the stomach has to be hot to produce a yellow moss.

If pale yellow (maybe white with yellow) it is still a normal tongue moss. However, if during the course of an outside evil the moss changes to yellow it indicates the disease is progressing inwards.

If moist it indicates an outside disease has just begun to go inside (e.g., the second stage of the six divisions) and the heat evil is not very strong.

If pasty and greasy it indicates internal heat and hot mucus.

If dry it indicates full internal heat.

If the root is yellow but the tip is white it indicates an outside evil just going inside or completely inside.

If the sides are yellow and the middle is white it indicates the patient has a tendency to be a little hot normally, or there is heat in the gall bladder and liver.

If the tip of the moss is yellow it indicates heat in the upper warmer.

If there are two yellow patches on the tongue, side by side longitudinally and the remainder of the moss is white it indicates the disease is still in the Tai Yang but beginning to go to Yang Ming.

(C) Black or Grey

This generally indicates a more serious disease. It may be due to extreme cold in the kidney or any other organs, or extreme heat so extreme that it appears like a cold disease. Dry moss indicates heat and wet moss indicates cold.

If thin greyish black (like a soot coating) it indicates cold and if an external condition then it implies coldness existed in the body prior to the external cold.

If only grey in the middle it indicates coldness in the spleen.

If moist and greasy it indicates a cold, damp, dirty evil in the intestines.

If thick and pasty it indicates cold damp mucus in the spleen.

If white with grey stripes it indicates a weak middle warmer or spleen allowing the cold to get in.

If white with black patches or spots it indicates damp heat inside or damp cold (dry = heat; wet = cold).

If white with black thorny appearance and dry it indicates internal heat and outside cold (Tai Yang is still cold and Yang Ming is hot). If moist it indicates cold both inside and outside.

If the centre is grey black and the edges white it indicates a cold problem of the middle heater (spleen yang weak).

If the centre is grey black and the edges and tip yellow and an outside condition, it indicates dry heat. If an inside condition, it indicates chronic damp heat.

If greasy and a soya sauce colour it indicates a chronic accumulation of damp heat in the middle heater.

4.25 Pulse Diagnosis

In traditional Chinese Medicine the pulses are classified into twenty eight qualities but the most important qualities are the following eight:

1. Floating

This pulse is felt on the superficial position and gives a sensation of floating on the surface of the skin.

It is associated with external symptoms which are caused by bacteria germs, virus, etc.

If the floating pulse is forceful it indicates a full external condition and denotes the over-powerful yang chi.

If the floating pulse is without force it indicates an empty external condition and denotes a deficiency of yin.

2. Deep

This pulse can only be felt in the deep position and gives a sensation of being sunken beneath the muscle. It is associated with internal symptoms. If the deep pulse is forceful it indicates a full internal condition and is a sign of an internal obstruction or stoppage.

If the deep pulse is without force it indicates an empty internal condition and denotes a deficiency of organic chi which means the function of the internal organs is weak.

3. Slow

The slow pulse has less than four beats during one respiration and generally indicates a cold condition. It is usually associated with a deep condition, and out of the yang divisions. It is an indication of weakness of the internal organs or lack of vitality due to this weakness.

If the slow pulse is forceful it indicates a full cold condition and denotes an internal chill and obstructions.

If the slow pulse is without force it indicates an empty cold condition and denotes the general weakness of the internal organs and a deficiency of yang.

4. Fast

The fast pulse has greater than five beats during one respiration and indicates an over abundance of heat (i.e., a hot condition) and yang chi. In serious cases the fast pulse is an indication of chi escaping from the body.

If the fast pulse is forceful it indicates a full hot condition and is a sign of internal heat or heat in the internal organs.

If the fast pulse is without force it indicates an empty hot condition and denotes general weakness of the body.

5. Slippery

This pulse is smooth and easy, like pearls rolling around a plate. It gives an impression of being flowing, round and slippery and will feel substantial under the fingers, probably stronger in the middle and lower levels. It indicates a disease due to mucus, or undigested food (i.e., weak stomach and spleen yang). If the slippery pulse is forceful it indicates mucus due to digestive problems.

If the slippery pulse is without force it indicates that the mucus is due to the weakness of the body.

6. **Rough or Choppy**
The quality of this pulse is the opposite of the slippery pulse. It is not fluent and lacks clean rhythm and amplitude. It can indicate empty blood, fluid loss, stuck cold dampness, or empty ching chi in the kidney.

If the rough pulse is forceful it indicates the disease is at a stationary stage and is difficult for the body to overcome (cold stuck dampness).

If the rough pulse is without force it indicates empty blood, weak organic function or empty ching chi.

7. **Empty**
This pulse has a floating and soft movement, and disappears on pressure.

It indicates empty blood or that the patient is very weak.

8. **Full**
This pulse gives an impression of being full, long and hard and responds to the finger strongly when pressed lightly or heavily. It is the opposite of the empty pulse.

It indicates an over abundance of heat dormant internally.

4.26 **General Body Signs**
Palpation of the abdomen and back should be performed with the purpose of identifying flaccid, hard, painful, bloated areas in relation to your knowledge of body areas controlled by particular organs.

Pain reflex on the mah (alarm) points should be determined, and also the shu points should be examined for heat, hardness or painful response. These examinations can identify problem organs and confirm other diagnostic signs.

Other general body areas which are said to be controlled by

particular organs should be observed for any abnormalities. Some of these body areas are as follows:

Feet

The transverse arch is controlled by the pericardium. Pericardium is deficient if the transverse arch is very thin.

The top of the foot is controlled by the stomach.

Bunched up toes indicates a colon problem.

Numb, cold and weak feet indicate a kidney problem.

Each of the toes is controlled by certain organs as follows:

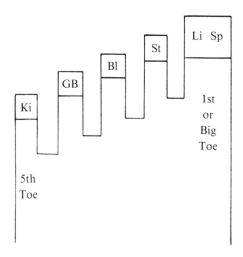

Ankle

The medial side of the ankle is controlled by the three heater and kidney.

The lateral side of the ankle is controlled by the gall bladder.

Knee

The knee is controlled by the kidney in general.

Above the knee belongs to metal.

Below the knee belongs to stomach.

Medial side of the knee belongs to liver and spleen.

Lateral side of the knee belongs to stomach and gall bladder.

Back of the knee belongs to bladder.

Hot knees indicate heat in the small intestine.

Cold knees indicate a deficient kidney.

Legs
The calves are controlled by the bladder and stomach.

The thigh muscles are controlled by the spleen.

Hip
The hip is controlled by the gall bladder and spleen.

Hands
The wrist belongs to the stomach.

Brown hands indicate a colon problem.

Damp hands indicate an earth problem.

Cold and limp indicate a water problem.

A mottled palm indicates a pericardium problem.

Dry hands indicate metal suppressing the pericardium.

A trembling ring finger indicates a three heater problem.

Elbow
Over extension of the elbow indicates a deficiency of the three heater, whereas under extension indicates excess of the three heater.

5. PHYSIOLOGY OF POINTS

Having formulated a treatment based on the diagnosis, it is important to know exactly what effects the chosen points may have. This can only be achieved if the practitioner has a thorough knowledge of each point. The following compendium of points indicates some considerations which should be made regarding point selection.

Bl 1 *Meridian Connections*
        GB
        Ht (Divergent)
        SI
        Sp (Divergent)
        St
        Yang Chiao Mo
        Yin Chiao Mo
        TH

        General Information
        Ht SI Upper Meeting point
        SI Bl (Tai Yang — Concentration point)
        SI Bl (Tai Yang — Meeting point)
        Sp St Upper Meeting point

    Indications
        Heat
            Cools heat.
        Meridian stagnation
            Moves the meridians.
        Wind
            Expels wind.

Bl10 *General Information*
Ki Bl Upper Meeting point
Sea of Energy with CV17 St 9
Window of the Sky point

Indications
Migraine
with GB20 and GB21.

Bl11 *Meridian Connections*
GB

General Information
Influential point for Bones
Sea of Blood with St37 St39

Bl12 *Meridian Connections*
GV

Indications
Asthma
Special point for Asthma.
Chi
Adjusts the chi.
Common Cold
Lungs
Assists in the circulation of Lu energy (used in the first stage of an external Lu problem).
Wind
Expels wind.

Bl13 *General Information*
Lu (Associated Effect Point – A.E.P.)

Indications
Chi
Regulates the chi.
Heat
Removes heat.
Lungs
Adjusts the Lu.

Bl14 *General Information*
Pe (A.E.P.)

Bl15   *General Information*
Ht (A.E.P.)

Indications
Blood
Regulates the blood (used in any Ht, blood or chi disorder).
Chi
Adjusts the chi (used in any Ht, blood or chi disorder).
Heart
Quietens the Ht (used in any Ht, blood or chi disorder).
Spirit or shen
Pacifies the spirit.

Bl17   *General Information*
Influential point for blood
Reunion point of yin and yang of the body.

Indications
Blood
Regulates the blood. Meeting point of all blood.
Emptiness
Tonifies emptiness.
Yang
Reunion point of yin and yang in the body.
Yin
Reunion point of yin and yang of the body.

Bl18   *General Information*
Li (A.E.P.)

Indications
Chi
Adjusts stuck chi.
Gall Bladder
Benefits the GB.
Heat
Cools damp heat (referring to jaundice or gastro intestinal problems).
Liver
Benefits the Li.

Bl19   *General Information*
GB (A.E.P.)

Indications
Chi
   Adjusts the chi.
Gall Bladder
   Cools, clears and disperses evil heat of the GB
   and Li.
Heat
   Cools, clears and disperses evil heat of the GB
   and Li.
Liver
   Cools, clears and disperses evil heat of the GB
   and Li.

Bl20   *General Information*
Sp (A.E.P.)

Indications
Blood
   Harmonizes the blood.
Dampness
   Expels water and dampness.
Spleen
   Adjusts Sp chi. Helps the transformation and
   moving aspects of the Sp. Therefore it is good
   for strengthening and unblocking or ensuring
   Sp energy is moving in the right direction.

Bl21   *General Information*
St (A.E.P.)

Indications
Dampness
   Transforms dampness.
Stomach
   Adjusts St Chi.

Bl22   *General Information*
TH (A.E.P.)

Indications
Chi
Adjusts the chi's transportation. Therefore good for any problems of empty metabolism.
Dampness
Benefits dampness and water (TH is in charge of waterways). Can be used as a diuretic to get rid of dampness.

Bl23 *Meridian Connections*
Ki (divergent)

General Information
Ki (A.E.P.)

Indications
Kidney
Adjusts Ki chi.

Bl24 *Indications*
Blood
Adjusts blood.
Chi
Adjusts chi.

Bl25 *General Information*
Co (A.E.P.)

Indications
Stomach
Adjusts the St.

Bl26 *Indications*
Dampness
Transforms stuck dampness in the lower heater (which shows as urinary symptoms).
Triple heater
Regulates the lower heater.

Bl27 *General Information*
SI (A.E.P.)

Indications
Dampness
  Benefits dampness.
Heat
  Cools heat.
Small intestine
  Moves and adjusts the St.

Bl28   *General Information*
Bl (A.E.P.)

Indications
Bladder
  Adjusts the Bl.

Bl30   *Indications*
Incontinence
  Incontinence of urine and faeces.
Quadraplegia

Bl31   *Meridian Connections*
GB

Indications
Fertility
  Infertility — both sexes.
Genitalia
  Genital diseases.
Hormones
  Hormonal imbalance.
Triple Heater
  Regulates the lower heater.

Bl32   *Indications*
Triple Heater
  Regulates the lower heater.

Bl33   *Meridian Connections*
GB

Indications
Triple Heater
  Regulates the lower heater.

Bl34   *Indications*
                Triple Heater
                    Regulates the lower heater.

Bl38   *Indications*
                Blood
                    Strengthens the blood.
                Emptiness
                    Tonifies emptiness and weakness.
                Lungs
                    Regulates Lu chi.

Bl50   *Indications*
                Haemorrhoids

Bl51   *Indications*
                Back problems
                    Difficulty in bending.
                Haemorrhoids

Bl53   *General Information*
                TH lower point

              Indications
                Bladder
                    Benefits the Bl.
                Fluid problems
                    Fluid retention. Don't use alone as will cause
                    fluid loss.

Bl54   *Meridian Connections*
                Ki (divergent)

              General Information
                Bl lower Ho point
                Ki Bl lower meeting point

              Indications
                Back problems
                    Back pain. Sciatica.
                Fluid problems
                    Fluid retention.

Heat
Disperses summer heat.
Leg problems
Sports injuries — calf muscles. With
Bl57,Bl60,Sp6,GB34.
Nausea
Obesity
Ulcers
Gastric and duodenal ulcers.

Bl57   *Indications*
Haemorrhoids
With GV1 and GV20.
Leg problems
Sports injuries. With Sp6, Bl54, GB34.

Bl58   *Indications*
Cystitis — Urogenital problems
With Ki3. Excessive use of Bl58 can cause
haemorrhoids.
Rheumatoid arthritis

Bl59   *Meridian Connections*
Yang Chiao Mo

General Information
Accumulation (Hung) point — Yang Chiao

Indications.
Facial problems — see also teeth problems
heavy feeling in head, facial paralysis.
Leg problems
Pain in thigh.
Quadraplegia

Bl60   *Indications*
Wind
Disperses wind in the head.

Bl61   *Meridian Connections*
Yang Chiao Mo

Bl62   *Meridian Connections*
Du Mo.   **Coupled Point**
Yang Chiao Mo. **Master Point**

Indications
Skin
Painful skin.
Spirit or shen
Clears and cools the spirit — has a very
strong effect on the spirit, hence good for
insomnia, epilepsy, etc.

Bl63   *Meridian Connections*
Yang Wei Mo

General Information
Accumulation (Hung) point

Indications
Abdomen
Lower abdominal pain.
Convulsion

Bl64   *Indications*
Spirit or shen
Calms the spirit.
Wind
Disperses wind.

Bl65   *Indications*
Skin
Skin problems. Abscesses.

Bl66   *Indications*
Headache — See migraine also

Bl67   *Meridian Connections*
Ki

General Information
SI Bl (Tai Yang — root point)

Indications
Labour
Difficult labour due to improperly positioned foetus.

Co 1   *Meridian Connections*
Lu

Indications
Facial problems — See also teeth problems toothache on opposite side of face.
Heat
Clears heat.
Skin
Acne on the face.
Teeth problems — See also facial problems toothache on opposite side of face.
Thyroid
Has direct affect on due to lung connection.
Wind
Controls wind caused by heat.

Co 2   *Indications*
Constipation
Massage also helpful.

Co 3   *Indications*
Hand problems
Red and swollen hands.

Co 3.5   *Indications*
Facial problems — See also teeth problems lower jaw analgesia.
Foot problems
Sore feet.

Co 4   *Indications*
Bronchitis
With Co1 and Lu11 on females.
Facial problems — See also teeth problems, face inflammation.

Hand problems
Sports injuries. with TH3, SI4, Pe6, TH6.
Meridian stagnation
Moves the face meridians.
Migraine
Sinus
With Co20.
Skin
Skin problems.
Sweating
Causes sweating (tonifies Wei chi).
Tonsils
Wind
Expels wind.

Co 5   *Indications*
Muscle — See limb problems etc.
Skin
Increases energy on skin surface.

Co 6   *Indications*
Breathing
Difficult or shallow breathing.
Chest
Tight chest.

Co 7   *General Information*
Accumulation (Hung) point

Indications
Abdomen
Abdominal pain. Intestinal noises.

Co10   *Indications*
Elbow problems
Tennis elbow.
Foot problems
Poor circulation to extremeties.
Hand problems
Poor circulation to extremeties.
Arthritis of hands and arms.
Paralysis
Hemiplegia.

Rheumatism
With St36 to tonify energy in cases of
rheumatism.

Co11   *General Information*
Co upper Ho point
Point of heaven, earth and man

Indications
Blood
Adjusts and harmonizes the blood and the
yung.
Blood pressure
With St36 — brings down blood pressure.
Dampness
Expels dampness in the intestines.
Depression
With Co4 for depression.
Elbow problems
Sports injuries. With Co10, Pe3, Lu5, Ht3.
Heat
Cools heat.
Indigestion
Parkinson's disease
Special point for Parkinson's disease (or any
shaking of extremeties.)
Skin
Dry skin.
Wind
Expels wind.

Co14   *Indications*
Meridian stagnation
Moves the meridians.

Co15   *Meridian Connections*
Yang Chiao Mo

Indications
Arm problems
Sports injuries. With Co11, Lu5, Ht3.
Chi
Circulates the chi.

Heat
Cools heat.
Meridian stagnation
Moves the meridians.
Shoulder problems
Sports injuries. With Co15, Co16, SI11, Co11.

Co16 *Meridian Connections*
Yang Chiao Mo

Indications
Blood
Moves stagnant blood (primarily in the chest region).
Meridian stagnation
Moves the meridians.

Co18 *General Information*
Lu Co upper meeting point
Window of the Sky point

Co20 *Meridian Connections*
St

General Information
Co St (Yang Ming — meeting point)

Indications
Lungs
Disperses wind heat in the Lu.

CV 1 *Meridian Connections*
Chong Mo
GV

General Information
Pe (alarm point) **no**

CV 1.5 *Indications*
Menopause
Menopause problems.

CV 2   *Meridian Connections*
GB (divergent)
Li

General Information
Li GB lower meeting point

Indications
Abdomen
Swollen Abdomen.
Chi
Yuan Chi affected (released) by this point.
Cystitis — Urogenital problems
Incontinence
Loss of bladder control.
Labour
Uterus returning to normal size after birth.

CV 3   *Meridian Connections*
Ki
Li
Sp

General Information
Bl (alarm point)

Indications
Chi
Benefits the transformation of chi through
the TH in general.
Yuan chi affected (released) by this point.
Cystitis — urogenital problems
Urogenital problems.
Gynaecological
Uterus prolapse.
Fibroids.
Heat
Benefits damp heat.
Impotence
Involuntary emissions. Weak erection.
Menstruation
Irregular periods.

CV 4 *Meridian Connections*
  Ki
  Li
  Sp

General Information
  Main tonification point for yang in the body.
  SI (alarm point)

Indications
  Abdomen
    Swollen abdomen.
  Chi
    Adjusts the chi (makes yang return).
  Cystitis – urogenital problems
    Urogenital problems.
  Gynaecological
    Retained placenta.
  Kidney
    Builds up to the Ki and firms up the body
    foundation.
  Rectum
    Rectum prolapse with GV1.
  Yang
    Main tonification point for the yang in the
    body.

CV 5 *General Information*
  TH (alarm point)

Indications
  Fertility
    Contraception point. Can cause sterility.

CV 6 *General Information*
  General source point for yin energy (lower yin).

Indications
  Chi
    Adjust the chi.
  Cystitis – Urogenital problems
    Urogenital problems.
  Fertility
    Lack of fertility.

Kidney
Tonifies the Ki.
Yin
General source point for lower yin energy.

CV 7   *Meridian Connections*
Chong Mo
Pe
TH

General Information
TH (alarm point)   no lower heater

Indications
Depression
Post-natal depression.

CV 8   *Indications*
Diarrhoea
Fatigue
Lactation deficiency
Stops excessive milk production.
Spleen
Strengthens the transforming power of the
Sp. The point of choice in problems of Sp
yang weak.
Stomach
Stomach ache.
Rids excess St gas.

CV 9   *Meridian Connections*
Lu

Indications
Edema

CV10   *Meridian Connections*
Sp

CV12   *Meridian Connections*
Li
Lu
Pe

SI
St
TH

General Information
  Influential point for yang organs
  Lu Sp (Tai Yin – concentration point)
  meeting point of 6 yang
  St (alarm point)
  TH (alarm point) ~~to~~ *middle heater*

Indications
  Appetite
    Lack of appetite.
  Blood pressure
    High blood pressure.
  Chi
    Regulates the chi and transforms the chi.
  Migraine
    With CV4 for migraine due to premenstrual tension.
  Stomach
    Adjusts the St.
  Ulcers
    Local point for ulcers.
  Vomiting
    Special point for vomiting.
  Yang
    Influential point for the yang organs.

CV13   *Meridian Connections*
  Lu
  SI
  St

CV14   *General Information*
  Ht (alarm point)

Indications
  Chi
    Adjusts the chi.
  Spirit or shen
    Calms the spirit.

Stomach
Harmonizes the St.

CV15 *General Information*
General source point for yin energy (upper yin)
Luo point of CV
Pe (alarm point) ᴺᵒ

Indications
Abdomen
Itchiness over abdomen.
Fatigue
Lack of energy in men (with GV19).
Managers disease.
Migraine
Smoking
Anti smoking.
Yin
General source point for upper yin energy.

CV17 *Meridian Connections*
Ki
Pe
SI
TH

General Information
Ht Ki (Shao yin – meeting point)
Influential point for energy
Sea of Energy with Bl10 St 9
P.C. TH (alarm point) *upper heater*

Indications
Asthma
Chi
Adjusts the chi.
Lactation deficiency
Insufficient milk.
Smoking
Plus ears-shenmen and 2Lu.
Anti smoking point (back up with shenmen
and Lu points).

CV18   *General Information*
Li Pe (Xue Yin – concentration point)

CV21   *Indications*
Asthma
Bronchitis

CV22   *Meridian Connections*
Yin Wei Mo

General Information
Window of the Sky point

Indications
Asthma
Massage if feel asthma attack coming on.
Special asthma point.
Bronchitis
Chi
Adjust the chi.
Facial problems – See also teeth problems
Swollen face. Lower jaw swollen. Toothache.
Needle towards bad side.
Hiccoughs
Moxa.
Lungs
Assists in the circulation function of the Lu.
Vagus
Has direct effect on vagus nerve.

CV22.5 *Indications*
Throat problems
Finger pressure for a few minutes will cure
sore throat.

CV23   *Meridian Connections*
Ki (divergent)
Pe (divergent)
Yin Wei Mo

General Information
Ht Ki (Shao Yin – Concentration point)

Indications.
Aphasia
Paralysis

CV24   *Meridian Connections*
Co
St

Indications
Vomiting
Prevents vomiting in females.

GB 1   *Meridian Connections*
Li (divergent)
SI
TH

General Information
GB TH (Shao Yang – meeting point)
Li GB upper meeting point

GB 2   *Indications*
Deafness
Tinnitus

GB 3   *Meridian Connections*
St

GB 4   *Meridian Connections*
St
TH

GB 5   *Meridian Connections*
St
TH

GB 6   *Meridian Connections*
St

GB 8   *Meridian Connections*
Bl

GB 9   *Meridian Connections*
Bl

GB10 *Meridian Connections*
Bl

GB11 *Meridian Connections*
Bl

GB12 *Meridian Connections*
Bl

GB13 *Meridian Connections*
Yang Wei Mo

Indications
Wind
Disperses wind.

GB14 *Meridian Connections*
Co
Yang Wei Mo
TH

GB15 *Meridian Connections*
Yang Wei Mo

GB16 *Meridian Connections*
Yang Wei Mo

GB17 *Meridian Connections*
Yang Wei Mo

GB18 *Meridian Connections*
Yang Wei Mo

GB19 *Meridian Connections*
Yang Wei Mo

GB20 *Meridian Connections*
Yang Chiao Mo
Yang Wei Mo

Indications
Common cold

Migraine
With GB21 and Bl10.
Wind
Moves wind. An important point for all wind
in the body whether internal or external.

GB21   *Meridian Connections*
Yang Wei Mo
TH

Indications
Hiccoughs
With SI15.
Neck problems – See shoulder problems
Sports injuries resulting in stiff neck.
With GB20,TH3 and special point between
2nd and 3rd metacarpals.

GB22   *Meridian Connections*
Ht (divergent)
Lu (divergent)
Pe (divergent)

General Information
Ht SI lower meeting point
Lu Co lower meeting point

GB23   *General Information*
GB (alarm point)

GB24   *Meridian Connections*
Sp
Yang Wei Mo

General Information
GB (alarm point)

GB25   *General Information*
Ki (alarm point)

GB26   *Meridian Connections*
Dai Mo

Indications
  Gynaecological
    Special gynaecological point.
  Heat
    Benefits damp heat, especially in the lower
    heater.

GB27 *Meridian Connections*
  Dai Mo

GB28 *Meridian Connections*
  Dai Mo

GB29 *Meridian Connections*
  Yang Chiao Mo

GB30 *Meridian Connections*
  Bl

  General Information
  Affects (releases) Yuan Chi.

  Indications
  Back problems
    Sciatica.
  Chi
    Yuan Chi affected (released) by this point.
  Leg problems
    Any problem of hip.

GB31 *Indications*
  Back problems
    Sciatica.
  Leg problems
    Arthritis of hip or knee.

GB33 *General Information*
  Accumulation (Hung) point – Yang Wei

GB34 *General Information*
  GB lower Ho point
  Influential point for muscles

Indications
Constipation
Gall Bladder
   Benefits the GB.
Heat
   Cools damp heat (all over the body).
Liver
   Benefits the Li.

GB35   *Meridian Connections*
Yang Wei Mo

Indications
Asthma
Chest
   Chest full and heavy.
Leg problems
   Neuralgia of leg.

GB36   *General Information*
Accumulation (Hung) point

Indications
Leg problems
   Calf spasm. Weakness and pain in leg.

GB37   *Indications*
Eyes
   Special point for eyes – with GB8.
Liver
   Adjusts and cools the Li.

GB39   *General Information*
Connects 3 lower yang
Group Luo point
Influential point for bone marrow.

Indications
Gall bladder
   Cools the GB.
Whiplash
   Use on opposite side.

Yang
    Connects the 3 lower yang.   Group Luo.

GB40   *Indications*
        Foot problems
            Red swollen heels.
        Liver
            Soothes and benefits the Li.

GB41   *Meridian Connections*
            Dai Mo   **Master Point**
            Yang Wei Mo. **Coupled Point**

        Indications
            Breast
                Breast ulcers.
            Foot problems
                Smelly feet.
            Gall bladder
                Disperses the Li and GB.
            Liver
                Disperses the Li and GB.
            Migraine
                Very useful for migraine.
            Sweating
                Excessive perspiration.

GB43   *Indications*
        Foot problems
            Tinea.

GB44   *General Information*
        GB TH (Shao Yang – root point)

GV 1   *Meridian Connections*
        GB
        Ki

        Indications
            Diarrhoea
            Haemorrhoids
                Bad haemorrhoids – GV1, GV20, Bl57.

Rectum
Rectum prolapse with GV20.

GV 2   *Indications*
Back problems
Lumbar neuralgia.
Haemorrhoids
Knee problems
Painful knees.

GV 3   *Indications*
Abdomen
Distended abdomen.
Back problems
Lumbago.
Cold
Expels cold damp.
Genitalia
Disturbances of genitals.
Kidney
Adjusts Ki chi.

GV 4   *Indications*
Chi
Builds up the original chi.
Deafness
Fatigue
Massage for general tonic in men.
Headache – See migraine also
headaches.
Kidney
Tonifies the Ki and Ki yang.

GV 8   *Indications*
Epilepsy
Heart
Cardiac pain.
Tension
Extreme tension – pent up anger.

GV 9   *Indications*
        Chi
            Regulates the chi.
        Dampness
            Transforms dampness.
        Hepatitis

GV10   *Indications*
        Back problems
            Back pain.
        Chest
            Chest pain.

GV12   *Indications*
        Lungs
            Lu problems.
        Tension
            Extreme tension.

GV14   *Meridian Connections*
        Bl
        Co
        GB
        SI
        St
        TH

        Indications
        Asthma
        Common cold
            Onset of colds with Co20.
        Cough
            Heavy cough.
        Fever
        Infection
        Paralysis
        Schizophrenia
        Shoulder problems
            Neck tension and shoulder problems.
        Skin
            Skin eruptions.
        Yang
            Meeting point of all the yang meridians.

GV15 *Meridian Connections*
Yang Wei Mo

General Information
Window of the Sky point

Indications
Concentration
Deafness
Deaf and dumb point.
Paralysis

GV16 *Meridian Connections*
Yang Wei Mo

General Information
Sea of bone marrow with GV20

Indications
Common cold
Post flu recovery.

GV17 *Meridian Connections*
Bl

GV19 *Indications*
Concentration
Dizziness

GV20 *Meridian Connections*
Bl
Li
TH (divergent)

General Information
Sea of bone marrow with GV16

Indications
Dizziness
Vertigo.
Epilepsy
Haemorrhoids
Headache – See migraine also
Insomnia

Liver
  Calms the Li (excess conditions) and
  extinguishes Li wind.
Rectum
  Rectal prolapse.
Shock
Spirit or shen
  Pacifies the spirit.

GV23 *Indications*
  Eyes
    Eye problems.
  Headache –See migraine also

GV24 *Meridian Connections*
  Bl
  St

GV24.5 *Indications*
  Dizziness
  Eyes
    Eye diseases.
  Migraine
  Sinus

GV25 *Indications*
  Alcoholism
    Sober up a drunk – stand behind him.

GV26 *Meridian Connections*
  Co
  St

  Indications
  Adrenals
    Actuates adrenals.
  Back problems
    Chronic back pain.
  Dribbling
  Kidney
    Kidney problems.
  Shock

GV27   *Indications*
              Teeth problems – See also facial problems
              Toothache.

GV28   *Meridian Connections*
              CV

Ht 1   *General Information*
              Ht SI lower meeting point

             Indications
              Paralysis
                Paralysis of all limbs.
              Sweating
                Excessive perspiration with general weakness.

Ht 3   *Indications*
              Depression
              Headache – See migraine also
                If due to wind.
              Spirit or shen
                Quietens the shen.

Ht 4   *Indications*
              Arthritis – elbow
              Hysteria
                With Ht1.
              Nervousness
                Calm with Ht,4,5,6,7.

Ht 5   *Indications*
              Fatigue
                Lack of energy, with SI4.
              Heart
                Adjusts Ht chi (use when pulse too slow).
              Spirit or shen
                Quietens the shen.

Ht 6   *General Information*
              Accumulation (Hung) point

             Indications
              Facial problems – See also teeth problems
                Epistaxis.

Headache – See migraine also
Suddenly mute with headache.
Palpitations
Sweating
Night sweats with SI3.

Ht 7   *Indications*
Depression
'Shenmen' – psychological problems.
Foot problems
Cold feet.
Hysteria
Insomnia
Due to over excitement.
Migraine
Palpitations
Spirit or shen
Pacifies the spirit (most important point for
the spirit).

Ht 8   *Indications*
Heart
Adjusts Ht chi.
Spirit or shen
Quietens the shen.

Ht 9   *Indications*
Heart
Tonifies Ht yin or yang.

Ki 1   *General Information*
Ht Ki (Shao Yin – root point)

Indications
Hysteria
Severe hysteria.
Incontinence
Inability to urinate.
Shock
Brings out of shock – will cause to cry and
urinate.

Ki 2   *Meridian Connections*
Yin Chiao Mo (only passes very near)

Indications
Diarrhoea
Impotence
Impotence. Sexual dysfunction.

Ki 3   *Indications*
Breast
Mammory pain.
Cough
With Lu10.
Fatigue
Weariness and fear.
Foot problems
Sports injuries. With Bl60, Li3, St44.
Sports injuries – ankle. With Bl60, GB3,
GB39, Sp5.
Hand problems
Cold hands.
Headache – See migraine also
Heat
Clears heat (more effective on empty heat).
Kidney
Benefits empty Ki yin.
Benefits the Ki.
Throat problems
Dry throat. Mouth and throat problems.

Ki 4   *Indications*
Depression
Inferiority complex – 'wishes to remain at
home'.
Menstruation
Painful menstruation and associated
emotional problems.

Ki 5   *General Information*
Accumulation (Hung) point

Indications
Depression
Depression.

Eyes
Myopia (near sightedness).
Gynaecological
Prolapsed uterus.
Menstruation
Premenstrual tension.
Shock
After slight shock.

Ki 6 *Meridian Connections*
Ren Mo   **Coupled Point**
Yin Chiao Mo **Master Point**

Indications
Heat
Clears heat.
Migraine
Due to premenstrual tension.
Shock
Emergency point for concussion and
unconsciousness.
Spirit or shen
Calms the spirit.
Stings
Massage for wasp, gnat and bee stings.

Ki 7 *Indications*
Cystitis – urogenital problems
Urogenital problems.
Fatigue
Extreme fatigue.
Foot problems
Cold feet.
Heat
Clears damp heat.
Kidney
Adjusts Ki chi and tonifies the Ki.
Knee problems
This point controls the knees.
Sweating
With Co4 for excessive sweating without
cause – will dry up in minutes.

Ki 8   *Meridian Connections*
Yin Chiao Mo

General Information
Accumulation (Hung) point – Yin Chiao

Indications
Genitalia
Swollen testes.
Gynaecological
Uterine bleeding.
Paralysis
Lower limb paralysis.

Ki 9   *Meridian Connections*
Yin Wei Mo

General Information
Accumulation (Hung) point – Yin Wei

Indications
Abdomen
Abdominal spasm in poisoning.
Epilepsy
Epilepsy and insanity.
Fertility
To promote conception – Ki9 on both mother
and father then Moxa Ki9 on mother in 3rd
and 6th month.
Foot problems
Painful feet.
Gynaecological
Gynaecological point.
Labour
Massage in 3rd and 6th month of pregnancy
to increase health of baby and its resistance to
disease.
Lactation deficiency
Leg problems
Weak legs.
Lymphatic
Moxa to drain lymphatic system.

Ki10   *Indications*
        Cystitis – urogenital problems
          Urogenital problems.
        Knee problems
          Moxa to strengthen weak knees.

Ki11   *Meridian Connections*
        Chong Mo

        General Information
        Pe (alarm point)

Ki12   *Meridian Connections*
        Chong Mo

        General Information
        SI Bl (Tai Yang – Shokanten point)

Ki13   *Meridian Connections*
        Chong Mo

Ki14   *Meridian Connections*
        Chong Mo

Ki15   *Meridian Connections*
        Chong Mo

Ki16   *Meridian Connections*
        Chong Mo

        General Information
        Ht Ki (Shao Yin – Shokanten point)

Ki17   *Meridian Connections*
        Chong Mo

Ki18   *Meridian Connections*
        Chong Mo

Ki19   *Meridian Connections*
        Chong Mo

        General Information
        Li Pe (Xue Yin – Shokanten point)

Ki20 *Meridian Connections*
Chong Mo

Ki21 *Meridian Connections*
Chong Mo

General Information
GB TH (Shao Yang – Shokanten point)

Li 1 *Meridian Connections*
GB

General Information
Li Pe (Xue Yin – root point)

Indications
Hernia
With Li4.

Li 2 *Indications*
Chi
Moves stuck chi.
Heat
Brings down fire.
Liver
Disperses the fire in the Li.
Menstruation
Irregular menses.

Li 3 *Indications*
Blood
Regulates the blood.
Blood pressure
With Li2 to bring down blood pressure –
+ Li3 − Li2.
Epilepsy
Gynaecological
Uterine bleeding.
Liver
Balances the Li. Very useful in empty Li yin
problems.

Li 4   *Indications*
Fluid problems
Generalized edema.
Incontinence
Urine retention.
Liver
Regulates the harmonizing effect of the Li.
Used particularly for a stuck condition of the
Li.

Li 5   *Indications*
Cystitis – urogenital problems
Urogenital problems, especially if
inflammation.

Li 6   *General Information*
Accumulation (Hung) point

Indications
Hernia
Leg problems
Leg pain.
Paralysis

Li 8   *Indications*
Bladder
Benefits the Bl.
Genitalia
Infection.
Heat
Cools and eliminates damp heat.
Impotence

Li10   *Indications*
Insomnia
Due to planning for tomorrow.

Li11   *Indications*
Insomnia

Li13   *Meridian Connections.*
Dai Mo
GB

General Information
Influential point for yin organs
Lu Sp (Tai Yin – Shokanten point)
Sp (alarm point)

Indications
Yin
Influential point for yin organs.

Li14   *Meridian Connections*
Sp
Yin Wei Mo

General Information
Li (alarm point)
Li Pe (Xue Yin – Shokanten point)

Indications
Chi
Soothes and benefits the chi.

Lu 1   *Meridian Connections*
Sp

General Information
Lu (alarm point)
Lu Sp (Tai Yin – meeting point)

Indications
Bronchitis
Lungs
All lung disorders.

Lu 2   *Meridian Connections*
Co (divergent)

Indications
Shoulder problems
Local point for shoulder neuralgia.

Lu 3   *General Information*
Window of the Sky point

Lu 5   *Indications*
            Chi
                Makes chi go down well.
            Cough
                Cough with thick dark mucus.
            Lungs
                Controls rebellion of chi in the Lu.
                Disperses heat in the Lu.
            Paralysis
                Hemiplegia.
            Quadraplegia

Lu 6   *General Information*
            Accumulation (Hung) point

            Indications
            Cough
                Cough with blood in phlegm.
            Heat
                Cools heat.
            Lungs
                Adjusts and sends down Lu energy.

Lu 7   *Meridian Connections*
            Ren Mo   **Master Point**
            Yin Chiao Mo   **Coupled Point**

            General Information
            Be careful using on females-can cause
            bronchitis. (Back with Co4 or Co11 to prevent).

            Indications
            Asthma
                With Co4 for asthma and migraine.
            Cough
            Lungs
                Circulates Lu energy in general.
            Throat problems
                Throat infection.
            Wind
                Disperses wind.

Yang
Takes energy out of the lung into the 6 yang.
General Luo.

Lu 8   *Indications*
Cough
Obstinate cough.

Lu 9   *General Information*
Influential point for pulses

Indications
Asthma
Asthma and wheezing.
Chi
Wei chi increased. Also anything that
depresses Li.
Cough
Dry cough.
Lungs
Regulates the Lu.
Mucus
Transforms mucus, and aids in the circulation
of damp sputum.
Wind
Disperses wind.

Lu10   *Indications*
Anxiety
Anxiety with palpitations.
Breast
Breast abscess.
Hand problems
Cold hands.
Lungs
Clears heat in the Lu.

Lu11   *Indications*
Chi
Aids in the circulation of energy.
Lungs
Cools the Lu.
Meningitis

Pe 1   *General Information*
  Li Pe (Xue Yin – meeting point)
  Pe (alarm point)
  Window of the Sky point

  Indications
  Breast
    Mammory pain.
  Lactation deficiency

Pe 3   *Indications*
  Blood
    Disperses hot blood.
  Cough
  Heart
    Moves Ht chi.
  Small intestine
    Adjusts the intestines.

Pe 4   *General Information*
  Accumulation (Hung) point

  Indications
  Chi
    Regulates the chi.
  Heart
    Ht pains of a muscular nature. Myocarditis.
    Quietens the Ht.
  Spirit or shen
    Calms the spirit.

Pe 5   *General Information*
  Group Luo point.

  Indications
  Mucus
    Expels mucus in the chest (Tan Yin obstructs
    the function of the Ht).
  Spirit or shen
    Calms the spirit.
  Stomach
    Harmonizes the St.
  Yin
    Balances upper yin.   Group Luo.

Pe 6   *Meridian Connections*
Chong Mo   **Coupled Point**

Indications
Chest
Feeling of heavy and tight chest.
Chi
Regulates the chi.
Depression
Psychological problems.
Heart
Calms the Ht.
Labour
Excessive bleeding after childbirth – with Sp
points. Nausea and vomiting in pregnancy.
Menstruation
Disturbed menses.
Nervousness
With TH5 for nervous breakdown.
Shock
Yang
Takes energy from all yin to the yang (this
balances yin yang on a large scale).
General Luo.

Pe 7   *Indications*
Breast
Painful breasts. Breast ulceration.
Chi
Regulates the chi.
Depression
Psychological problems.
Lymphatic
Lymphatic problems – with Sp points.
Spirit or shen
Quietens the spirit.
Stomach
Harmonizes the St.

Pe 8   *General Information*
Pe (alarm point)

Indications
Hand problems
Sweaty palms. Hand disorders. Cold hands
due to circulatory problems.
Heart
Cools the Ht.
Heat
Disperses heat.

Pe 9 *Indications*
Fever
Fever without sweating – induces sweating.
Sweating
Induces sweating.
Tinnitus

SI 1 *Indications*
Headache – See migraine also
Head neuralgias. Headache with diarrhoea
together.
Heat
Disperses wind heat.
Lactation deficiency
Shock

SI 2 *Indications*
Fever
Fever when no sweating if confirmed by
pulses.
Tinnitus

SI 3 *Meridian Connections*
Du Mo **Master Point**
Yang Chiao Mo **Coupled Point**

General Information
Main source point for all of the body and
meridians.

Indications
Shock
Slow recovery from shock.

Shoulder problems
Shoulder pain. Shoulder relaxation. Twisted
back on opposite side.
Tension

SI 4 *Indications*
Sweating
Use with Ki7 for excessive sweating.

SI 5 *Indications*
Dizziness
Use with discretion.

SI 6 *General Information*
Accumulation (Hung) point

Indications
Arm problems
Paralysis of arm.
Eyes
Bloodshot and congested eyes.

SI 7 *Indications*
Anxiety
Throat problems
Acute throat pain.

SI 8 *General Information*
SI upper Ho point

SI10 *Meridian Connections*
Yang Chiao Mo
Yang Wei Mo

SI11 *Indications*
Arthritis – arm, shoulder – See shoulder
problems

SI12 *Meridian Connections*
Co
GB
TH

Indications
Angina

SI16 *General Information*
Window of the Sky point

SI17 *General Information*
Window of the Sky point

Indications
Tonsils
With Co4.

SI18 *Meridian Connections*
GB
TH

SI19 *Meridian Connections*
GB
TH

Indications
Deafness
Tinnitus
Trigeminal Neuralgia

Sp 1 *Meridian Connections*
St

General Information
Lu Sp (Tai Yin – root point)

Indications
Abortion
Use Sp1,3,4,6 and Co4.
Blood
Adjusts the blood and is especially used to
hold blood in the meridians.
Foot problems
Foot paralysis.
Cold feet.
Shock
Good for use after shock.
Spleen
Benefits the Sp.

Sp 2   *Indications*
Bunions
With Sp3, Li2. Treat each day for 5 days then rest for 3 and repeat if necessary.
Mucus
Expels mucus caused by weak Sp (i.e., Sp sending up dirty energy to the Lu).
Spleen
Tonifies the Sp.

Sp 3   *Indications*
Diarrhoea
Diarrhoea with blood.
Shock
Eliminates post trauma shock (especially with amnesia) – i.e., after affects of shock due to bad memories.

Sp 4   *Meridian Connections*

| Chong Mo | **Master Point** |
| Yin Wei Mo | **Coupled Point** |

Indications
Genitalia
Injury to testicles.
Indigestion
Key point in digestive diseases.
Labour
Stretch marks after pregnancy.

Sp 5   *Indications*
Fertility
Sterility.
Joints
Dislocated joints.
Loose joints (Moxa more affective).
Spleen
Strengthens the Sp and St.
Strengthens Sp yang in general.
Stomach
Strengthens the Sp and St.

Sp 6   *Meridian Connections*
      Ki
      Li

      General Information
      Group Luo point

      Indications
      Dampness
        Transforms dampness.
      Depression
        Nervous depression.
      Diarrhoea
      Endocrine
      Gynaecological
        With Co6 for internal inflammations and
        ulceration of uterus etc. (also Co11).
      Impotence
        Frigidity – Sp6, CV4, Bl23, Bl54, CV3, ear
        shenmen.
        Sexual problems.
      Indigestion
      Insomnia
      Kidney
        Strengthens the Ki.
      Liver
        Opens up and softens the Li.
      Menstruation
        Menstruation regulation with Pe6. With Co4
        for bringing on period.
      Pancreas
      Spleen
        Strengthens the Sp.
      Stomach
        Gastro Intestinal disorders with St36.
      Thyroid
      Yin
        Meeting point of 3 lower yin.

Sp 8   *General Information*
      Accumulation (Hung) point

Indications
Blood
Regulates the blood (good for empty blood or blood running out of course).
Gynaecological
Special urogenital point for uterus problems. Special point.
Menstruation
Painful menses.

Sp 9 *Indications*
Dampness
Transforms stuck dampness (also strengthens the lower Htr).
Edema
Fluid problems
With Sp4 to rid excess fluids.
Haemorrhoids
Leg problems
Weak legs.
Sports injuries. Good for knee and muscle injuries around area.
Menstruation
Menstrual problems.

Sp10 *Indications*
Allergy
Blood
Harmonizes and cools the blood. Use moxa to tonify the blood.
Special point for blood disorders.
Menstruation
Irregular periods.
Skin
2 up is special skin point (nest of 100 caterpillars) with Co11.

Sp11 *Indications*
Muscle – See limb problems etc.
Sports injuries. Muscular injuries with Sp10, Sp6. Bl60 for pain.

Sp12   *Meridian Connections*
    Li

    General Information
    Affects (releases) Yuan Chi

    Indications
    Chi
      Yuan Chi affected (released) by this point.

Sp13   *Meridian Connections*
    Li
    Yin Wei Mo

Sp15   *Meridian Connections*
    Yin Wei Mo

Sp16   *Meridian Connections*
    Yin Wei Mo

Sp21   *General Information*
    Balances left and right, and internal and external.
    Great Luo of spleen
    Lu Sp (Tai Yin – Shokanten point)

St 1   *Meridian Connections*
    Co
    CV
    Li
    Yang Chiao Mo

    General Information
    Sp St upper meeting point

St 2   *Indications*
    Gall bladder
      Benefits the GB.
    Liver
      Assists the Li in its dispersing function.
    Wind
      Expels wind.

St 3   *Meridian Connections*
Yang Chiao Mo

St 4   *Meridian Connections*
Yang Chiao Mo

Indications
Facial problems – See also teeth problems
Mouth problems (e.g., ulcers).

St 5   *Meridian Connections*
GB

Indications
Facial problems – See also teeth problems
Facial acne.
Skin
Facial acne.
Teeth problems – See also facial problems
Local point for toothache.

St 6   *Meridian Connections*
GB

Indications
Facial problems – See also teeth problems
Facial Neuralgia.
Meridian Stagnation
Moves the meridians.
Wind
Expels wind.

St 7   *General Information*
Co St (Yang Ming – concentration point)

St 8   *Indications*
Headache – See migraine also
With St34.

St 9   *General Information*
Sea of Energy with CV17 Bl10
Window of the Sky point

Indications
Blood
Adjusts blood.
Chi
Adjusts chi.

St12 *Meridian Connections*
Co
GB
Lu (divergent)
SI
Yin Chiao Mo
TH

Indications
Vomiting
Prevents vomiting (particularly in male).
Good for nausea and vomiting due to dialysis
machine.

St18 *Indications*
Lactation deficiency

St25 *Meridian Connections*
Co

General Information
Co (alarm point)
GB TH (Shao Yang – Shokanten point)

Indications
Chi
Regulates chi and reduces stuckness generally
in the lower abdominal area.
Diarrhoea
With Bl25 – if doesn't work then really sick.

St27 *General Information*
Co St (Yang Ming – Shokanten point)

St28 *Indications*
Bladder
Benefits the Bl.

Heat
Clears damp heat in the lower part of the
body (e.g., discharge or hot damp diarrhoea).

St29   *Indications*
Prostate
Prostate and Gonads.

St30   *Meridian Connections*
Chong Mo
GB
Sp (divergent)

General Information
Affects (releases) Yuan chi.
Sea of Nourishment with St36
Sp St lower meeting point

Indications
Chi
Yuan chi affected (released) by this point.
Menopause
Menopausal problems.

St31   *Indications*
Muscle – see limb problems etc.
Strained thigh muscles – footballers injuries.
St31,St36, St44. Sedate if heavy drainage of
energy. Also use Co4 as a supplement. GB34.
Bl60 for pain.

St34   *General Information*
Accumulation (Hung) point

Indications
Meridian stagnation
Moves the St meridian (therefore indicated for
leg problems).
Stomach
Gastralgia.
Harmonizes the St in excess conditions.

St35 *Indications*
  Knee problems
    Local point for arthritic knees (and Bl54).

St36 *General Information*
  Sea of Nourishment with St30
  St lower Ho point

  Indications
  Blood
    Adjusts blood in general.
  Chi
    Wei chi increased. Also anything that
    depresses Li.
    Adjusts chi in general.
  Constipation
    Excessive use may cause constipation.
  Diarrhoea
    Excessive use may cause constipation.
  Impotence
    Sexual problems due to lack of energy.
  Indigestion
    Severe indigestion or acidity.
  Knee problems
    Sports injuries. St36 to reduce swelling. Li3
    for muscles.
    Bl60 for pain. St35 knee, eyes. GB34 for
    muscular problems.
    Bl54. Crane wind. GB31.
  Spleen
    Regulates the Sp.
  Stomach
    Regulates the St.

St37 *General Information*
  Co Lower Ho point
  Sea of Blood with Bl11 St39

  Indications
  Chi
    Assists in the downward movement of chi,
    and in general moves stuckness.

Heat
Cools damp heat.
Stomach
Regulates the St.

St38   *Indications*
Shoulder problems
Frozen shoulder – often immediate results.

St39   *General Information*
Sea of Blood with Bl11 St37
SI lower Ho point

St40   *Indications*
Alcoholism
Dampness
General point for all dampness problems as it
transforms dampness.
Depression
Nervous depression.
Leg problems
Leg paralysis.
Migraine
Mucus
General point for all mucus problems as it
transforms mucus.
Talking
Stops people continually talking.

St41   *Indications*
Facial problems – See also teeth problems
Facial paralysis.
Stomach
Tonifies the St.
Cold Damp stomach (indigestion from unripe
fruit) – warms the stomach.

St42   *Indications*
Facial problems – See also teeth problems
Facial paralysis.
Foot problems
Dropped foot – add St36 and Moxa Sp5.

Teeth problems – See also facial problems

St43   *Indications*
Belching
Fever
Indigestion
Indigestion and excessive thirst.

St44   *Indications*
Appetite
Loss of appetite.
Chi
Regulates chi.
Facial problems – See also teeth problems
Lower jaw problems. Anaesthetic for dental
work.
Foot problems
With GB34 and Co11 to relieve cold hands
and feet.
Hand problems
With GB34 and Co11 to relieve cold hands
and feet.
Hangovers
Before and after drinking to minimize
hangover.
Heat
Disperses heat.
Throat problems
Sore throat.

St45   *General Information*
Co St (Yang Ming – root point)

Indications
Cold
Disperses cold.
Edema
Facial problems – See also teeth problems
St45-42 for mouth afflictions (e.g.,
toothache).
Fullness
Disperses fullness (mostly for full hot
conditions).

Heat
Disperses heat.
Insomnia
Insomnia after a heavy meal.
Teeth problems – See also facial problems
St45-42 for mouth afflictions (e.g.,toothache).

Tai Yang   *General Information*
GB TH (Shao Yang – concentration point)

TH 1   *Meridian Connections*
Pe

Indications
Fatigue
Exhaustion. Summer heat diseases.

TH 2   *Indications*
Foot problems
Icy cold limbs.
Hand problems
Icy cold limbs.
Tinnitus

TH 3   *Indications*
Chi
Disperses and softens the chi.
Headache – See migraine also
with SI3.
Migraine
Shoulder problems
Back and shoulder problems.
Tinnitus

TH 4   *Indications*
Heat
Removes heat.
Triple heater
Moves the Meridian.

TH 5 *Meridian Connections*
  Dai Mo   **Coupled Point**
  Yang Wei Mo **Master Point**

 Indications
  Arthritis – arm, shoulder – See shoulder
  problems
   Arthritis of upper limb.
  Chi
   Wei chi increased. Also anything that
   depresses Li.
  Heat
   Liberates heat.
  Meridian stagnation
   Moves the meridians and stuck chi. Moves the
   yang of the body.
  Yin
   Takes energy from all the yang to the yin (this
   balances yin and yang on a large scale).
   General Luo.

TH 6 *Indications*
  Blood
   Disperses stuck blood.
  Chi
   Circulates the chi.
  Constipation
  Depression
  Labour
   Excessive bleeding after childbirth.
  Pleurisy

TH 7 *General Information*
  Accumulation (Hung) point

 Indications
  Chi
   Blocked chi as in a chronic disease.
  Nervousness
   Nervous trembling.

TH 8 *General Information*
  Group Luo point.

Meeting point for yang in the upper part of the body.

Indications
Fatigue
Good for lethargy.
Meridian stagnation
Moves and opens up the upper yang meridians. TH8 is the meeting point for yang in the upper part of the body.
Yang
Meeting point for yang in the upper part of the body. Moves and opens up the upper yang meridians.   Group Luo.

TH10   *General Information*
TH upper Ho point

Indications
Headache – See migraine also
Sweating
Excessive perspiration.

TH11   *Indications*
Shoulder problems

TH13   *Meridian Connections*
Co

TH14   *Indications*
Shoulder problems

TH15   *Meridian Connections*
Yang Wei Mo

Indications
Headache – See migraine also
weather point.

TH16   *General Information*
Pe TH upper meeting point
Window of the Sky point

TH17 *Meridian Connections*
    GB
    SI

    Indications
    Deafness
    Mumps
    Tinnitus
    Wind
      Disperses wind.

TH19 *Indications*
    Vomiting
      Vomiting in children.

TH20 *Meridian Connections*
    GB

TH21 *Indications*
    Deafness
    Heat
      Disperses evil heat locally.
    Tinnitus

Notes and definition of terminologies.

'Adjusts'	– A point adjusts if it clears obstructions (stuckness) and is used for energy going in opposition to its direction.
'Benefits'	– Strengthens.
'Moves the meridians'	– These points are indicated in circulation problems within a meridian.
'Opens'	– Encourages circulation of.
'Regulates'	– These points are effective in areas of stuckness and opposition, and tonify emptiness.
Regulation of organs	– A good rule is AEP + source.

6. INDICATION REFERENCE

Abdomen
Bl 63	Lower abdominal pain.
Co 7	Abdominal pain. Intestinal noises.
CV 2	Swollen abdomen.
CV 4	Swollen abdomen.
CV15	Itchiness over abdomen.
GV 3	Distended abdomen.
Ki 9	Abdominal spasm in poisoning.

Abortion
Sp 1	Use Sp1,3,4,6 and Co4.

Adrenals
GV26	Actuates adrenals.

Alcoholism
GV25	Sober up a drunk – stand behind him.
St40	

Allergy
Sp10

Angina
SI12

Anxiety
Lu10	Anxiety with palpitations.
SI 7	

Aphasia
    CV23

Appetite
    CV12   Lack of appetite.
    St44   Loss of appetite.

Arm problems
    Co15   Sports injuries. With Co11, Lu5,
                    Ht3.
    SI 6   Paralysis of arm.

Arthritis – Arm,   Shoulder – See shoulder problems.
    SI11
    TH 5   Arthritis of upper limb.

Arthritis – Elbow
    Ht 4

Asthma
    Bl 12   Special point for asthma.
    CV17
    CV21
    CV22   Massage if feel asthma attack coming
                    on.
                    Special asthma point.
    GB35
    GV14
    Lu 7   With Co4 for asthma and migraine.
    Lu 9   Asthma and wheezing.

Back problems
    Bl 51   Difficulty in bending.
    Bl 54   Back pain. Sciatica.
    GB30   Sciatica.
    GB31   Sciatica.
    GV 2   Lumbar neuralgia.
    GV 3   Lumbago.
    GV10   Back pain.
    GV26   Chronic back pain.

Belching
St43

Bladder

Bl 28	Adjusts the Bl.
Bl 53	Benefits the Bl.
Li 8	Benefits the Bl.
St28	Benefits the Bl.

Blood

Bl 15	Regulates the blood (used in any Ht, blood or chi disorder).
Bl 17	Regulates the blood. Meeting point of all blood.
Bl 20	Harmonizes the blood.
Bl 24	Adjusts blood.
Bl 38	Strengthens the blood.
Co11	Adjusts and harmonizes the blood and the Yung.
Co16	Moves stagnant blood (primarily in the chest region).
Li 3	Regulates the blood.
Pe 3	Disperses hot blood.
Sp 1	Adjusts the blood and is especially used to hold blood in the meridians.
Sp 8	Regulates the blood (good for empty blood or blood running out of course).
Sp10	Harmonizes and cools the blood. Use moxa to tonify the blood. Special point for blood disorders.
St 9	Adjusts blood.
St36	Adjusts blood in general.
TH 6	Disperses stuck blood.

Blood pressure

Co11	With St36 – brings down blood pressure.
CV12	High blood pressure.
Li 3	With Li2 to bring down blood pressure – +Li3 −Li2.

Breast

GB41	Breast ulcers.
Ki 3	Mammory pain.
Lu10	Breast abscess.
Pe 1	Mammory pain.
Pe 7	Painful breasts. Breast ulceration.

Breathing

Co 6	Difficult or shallow breathing.

Bronchitis

Co 4	With Co1 and Lu11 on females.
CV21	
CV22	
Lu 1	

Bunions

Sp 2	With Sp3, Li2. Treat each day for 5 days then rest for 3 and repeat if necessary.

Chest

Co 6	Tight chest.
GB35	Chest full and heavy.
GV10	Chest pain.
Pe 6	Feeling of heavy and tight chest.

Chi

	Formula to increase chi – St36,37,39 Co6 to 10, St30,36.
Bl 12	Adjusts the chi.
Bl 13	Regulates the chi.
Bl 15	Adjusts the chi (used in any Ht, blood or chi disorder).
Bl 18	Adjusts stuck chi.
Bl 19	Adjusts the chi.
Bl 22	Adjusts the chi's transportation. Therefore good for any problems of empty metabolism.
Bl 24	Adjusts chi.
Co15	Circulates the chi.
CV 2	Yuan Chi affected (released) by this point.

CV 3	Benefits the transformation of chi through the TH in general. Yuan Chi affected (released) by this point.
CV 4	Adjusts the chi (makes yang return).
CV 6	Adjusts the chi.
CV12	Regulates the chi and transforms the chi.
CV14	Adjusts the chi.
CV17	Adjusts the chi.
CV22	Adjusts the chi.
GB30	Yuan chi affected (released) by this point.
GV 4	Builds up the original chi.
GV 9	Regulates the chi.
Li 2	Moves stuck chi.
Li14	Soothes and benefits the chi.
Lu 5	Makes chi go down well.
Lu 9	Wei Chi increased. Also anything that depresses Li.
Lu11	Aids in the circulation of energy.
Pe 4	Regulates the chi.
Pe 6	Regulates the chi.
Pe 7	Regulates the chi.
Sp12	Yuan chi affected (released) by this point.
St 9	Adjusts chi.
St25	Regulates chi and reduces stuckness generally in the lower abdominal area.
St30	Yuan chi affected (released) by this point.
St36	Adjusts chi in general. Wei Chi increased. Also anything that depresses Li.
St37	Assists in the downward movement of chi, and in general moves stuckness.
St44	Regulates chi.
TH 3	Disperses and softens the chi.
TH 5	Wei chi increased. Also anything that depresses Li.

TH 6	Circulates the chi.
TH 7	Blocked chi as in a chronic disease.

Cold

GV 3	Expels cold damp.
St45	Disperses cold.

Common cold

Bl12	
GB20	
GV14	Onset of colds with Co20.
GV16	Post flu recovery.

Concentration

GV15
GV19

Constipation

Co 2	Massage also helpful.
GB34	
St36	Excessive use may cause constipation.
TH 6	

Convulsion

Bl 63

Cough

GV14	Heavy cough.
Ki 3	With Lu10.
Lu 5	Cough with thick dark mucus.
Lu 6	Cough with blood in phlegm.
Lu 7	
Lu 8	Obstinate cough.
Lu 9	Dry cough.
Pe 3	

Cystitis – urogenital problems

Bl 58	With Ki3. Excessive use of Bl 58 can cause haemorrhoids.
CV 2	

CV 3	Urogenital problems.
CV 4	Urogenital problems.
CV 6	Urogenital problems.
Ki 7	Urogenital problems.
Ki10	Urogenital problems.
Li 5	Urogenital problems, especially if inflammation.

Dampness

Bl 20	Expels water and dampness.
Bl 21	Transforms dampness.
Bl 22	Benefits dampness and water (TH is in charge of waterways). Can be used as a diuretic to get rid of dampness.
Bl 26	Transforms stuck dampness in the lower heater (which shows as urinary symptoms).
Bl 27	Benefits dampness.
Co11	Expels dampness in the intestines.
GV 9	Transforms dampness.
Sp 6	Transforms dampness.
Sp 9	Transforms stuck dampness (also strengthens the lower heater).
St40	General point for all dampness problems as it transforms dampness.

Deafness

GB 2	
GV 4	
GV15	Deaf and dumb point.
SI19	
TH17	
TH21	

Depression

Co11	With Co4 for depression.
CV 7	Post natal depression.
HT 3	
HT 7	'Shenmen' – psychological problems
Ki 4	Inferiority complex – 'wishes to remain at home'.
Ki 5	Depression.

Pe 6	Psychological problems.
Pe 7	Psychological problems.
Sp 6	Nervous depression.
St40	Nervous depression.
TH 6	

Diarrhoea

CV 8	
GV 1	
Ki 2	
Sp 3	Diarrhoea with blood
Sp 6	
St25	With Bl 25 – if doesn't work then really sick.
St36	Excessive use may cause constipation.

Dizziness

GV19	
GV20	Vertigo.
GV24.5	
SI 5	Use with discretion.

Dribbling

GV26

Edema

CV 9
Sp 9
St45

Elbow problems

| Co10 | Tennis elbow. |
| Co11 | Sports injuries. With Co10, Pe3, Lu5, Ht3. |

Emptiness

	Use local points
Bl 17	Tonifies emptiness.
Bl 38	Tonifies emptiness and weakness.

Endocrine

Sp 6

Epilepsy

GV 8	
GV20	
Ki 9	Epilepsy and insanity.
Li 3	

Eyes

GB37	Special point for eyes – with GB8.
GV23	Eye problems.
GV24.5	Eye diseases.
Ki 5	Myopia (near sightedness).
SI 6	Bloodshot and congested eyes.

Facial problems – see also teeth problems

Bl 59	Heavy feeling in head. Facial paralysis.
Co 1	Toothache on opposite side of face.
Co 3.5	Lower jaw analgesia.
Co 4	Face inflammation.
CV22	Swollen face. Lower jaw swollen. Toothache. Needle towards bad side.
Ht 6	Epistaxis.
St 4	Mouth problems (e.g., ulcers).
St 5	Facial acne.
St 6	Facial neuralgia.
St41	Facial paralysis.
St42	Facial paralysis.
St44	Lower jaw problems. Anaesthetic for dental work.
St45	St45-42 for mouth afflictions (e.g., toothache).

Fatigue

CV 8	
CV15	Lack of energy in men (with GV19). Managers disease.
GV 4	Massage for general tonic in men.
Ht 5	Lack of energy, with SI4.
Ki 3	Weariness and fear.
Ki 7	Extreme fatigue.
TH 1	Exhaustion. Summer heat diseases.
TH 8	Good for lethargy.

Fertility

Bl 31	Infertility – both sexes.
CV 5	Contraception point. Can cause sterility.
CV 6	Lack of fertility.
Ki 9	To promote conception – Ki 9 on both mother and father then moxa Ki 9 on mother in 3rd and 6th month.
Sp 5	Sterility.

Fever

GV14	
Pe 9	Fever without sweating – induces sweating.
SI 2	Fever when no sweating if confirmed by pulses.
St43	

Fluid problems

Bl 53	Fluid retention. Don't use alone as will cause fluid loss.
Bl 54	Fluid retention.
Li 4	Generalized edema.
Sp 9	With Sp4 to rid excess fluids.

Foot problems

Co 3.5	Sore feet.
Co10	Poor circulation to extremeties.
GB 40	Red swollen heels.
GB 41	Smelly feet.
GB 43	Tinea.
Ht 7	Cold feet.
Ki 3	Sports injuries – ankle. With Bl 60, GB3, GB39, Sp5. Sports injuries. With Bl 60, Li3, St44.
Ki 7	Cold feet.
Ki 9	Painful feet.
Sp 1	Cold feet. Foot paralysis.
St42	Dropped foot – add St36 and moxa Sp5.

St44	With GB34 and Co11 to relieve cold hands and feet.
TH 2	Icy cold limbs.

Fullness

Use distal points

St45	Disperses fullness (mostly for full hot conditions).

Gall Bladder

Bl 18	Benefits the GB.
Bl 19	Cools clears and disperses evil heat of the GB and Li.
GB34	Benefits the GB.
GB39	Cools the GB.
GB41	Disperses the Li and GB.
St 2	Benefits the GB.

Genitalia

Bl 31	Genital diseases.
GV 3	Disturbances of genitals.
Ki 8	Swollen testes.
Li 8	Infection.
Sp 4	Injury to testicles.

Gynaecological

CV 3	Fibroids.
	Uterus prolapse.
CV 4	Retained placenta.
GB26	Special gynaecological point.
Ki 5	Prolapsed uterus.
Ki 8	Uterine bleeding.
Ki 9	Gynaecological point.
Li 3	Uterine bleeding.
Sp 6	With Co6 for internal inflammations and ulceration of uterus etc. (also Co11).
Sp 8	Special point. Special urogenital point for uterus problems.

Haemorrhoids

Bl 50	
Bl 51	
Bl 57	With GV1 and GV20.
GV 1	Bad haemorrhoids – GV1, GV20, Bl 57.
GV 2	
GV20	
Sp 9	

Hand problems

Co 3	Red and swollen hands.
Co 4	Sports injuries. With TH3, SI4, Pe6, TH6.
Co10	Arthritis of hands and arms. Poor circulation to extremeties.
Ki 3	Cold hands.
Lu10	Cold hands.
Pe 8	Sweaty palms. Hand disorders. Cold hands due to circulatory problems.
St44	With GB34 and Co11 to relieve cold hands and feet.
TH 2	Icy cold limbs.

Hangovers

St44	Before and after drinking to minimize hangover.

Headache – see migraine also

Bl 66	
GV 4	Headaches.
GV20	
GV23	
Ht 3	If due to wind.
Ht 6	Suddenly mute with headache.
Ki 3	
SI 1	Head neuralgias. Headache with diarrhoea together.
St 8	With St34.
TH 3	With SI3.
TH10	
TH15	Weather point.

Heart

Bl 15	Quietens the Ht (used in any Ht, blood or chi disorder).
GV 8	Cardiac pain.
Ht 5	Adjusts Ht chi (use when pulse too slow).
Ht 8	Adjusts Ht chi.
Ht 9	Tonifies Ht yin or yang.
Pe 3	Moves Ht chi.
Pe 4	Ht pains of a muscular nature. Myocarditis. Quietens the Ht.
Pe 6	Calms the Ht.
Pe 8	Cools the Ht.

Heat

Bl 1	Cools heat.
Bl 13	Removes heat.
Bl 18	Cools damp heat (referring to jaundice or gastro intestinal problems).
Bl 19	Cools clears and disperses evil heat of the GB and Li.
Bl 27	Cools heat.
Bl 54	Disperses summer heat.
Co 1	Clears heat.
Co11	Cools heat.
Co15	Cools heat.
CV 3	Benefits damp heat.
GB26	Benefits damp heat, especially in the lower heater.
GB34	Cools damp heat (all over the body).
Ki 3	Clears heat (more effective on empty heat).
Ki 6	Clears heat.
Ki 7	Clears damp heat.
Li 2	Brings down fire.
Li 8	Cools and eliminates damp heat.
Lu 6	Cools heat.
Pe 8	Disperses heat.
SI 1	Disperses wind heat.
St28	Clears damp heat in the lower part of the body (e.g., discharge or hot damp diarrhoea).

St37	Cools damp heat.
St44	Disperses heat.
St45	Disperses heat.
TH 4	Removes heat.
TH 5	Liberates heat.
TH21	Disperses evil heat locally.

Hepatitis

Tonify earth. Sedate water. Sedate wood.

GV 9

Hernia
| Li 1 | With Li4. |
| Li 6 | |

Hiccoughs
| CV22 | Moxa. |
| GB21 | With SI15. |

Hormones
| Bl 31 | Hormonal imbalance. |

Hysteria
Ht 4	With Ht1.
Ht 7	
Ki 1	Severe hysteria.

Impotence

Check Ki, Li, Sp.

CV 3	Involuntary emissions. Weak erection.
Ki 2	Impotence. Sexual dysfunction.
Li 8	
Sp 6	Frigidity – Sp6, CV4, Bl 23, Bl 54, CV3, ear shenmen. Sexual problems.
St36	Sexual problems due to lack of energy.

Incontinence

Bl 30	Incontinence of urine and faeces.
CV 2	Loss of bladder control.
Ki 1	Inability to urinate.
Li 4	Urine retention.

Indigestion

Co11	
Sp 4	Key point in digestive diseases.
Sp 6	
St36	Severe indigestion or acidity.
St43	Indigestion and excessive thirst.

Infection

GV14

Inflammation

Use distal points

Insomnia

Types: Weakness of Ht and St.
Functional disconnection of Li and GB.
Yin yang disturbance of Sp and St.
Good points: Ht7, Co4, St36, Sp6, Pe6, Li2.

GV20	
HT 7	Due to over excitement.
Li10	Due to planning for tomorrow.
Li11	
Sp 6	
St45	Insomnia after a heavy meal.

Joints

Sp 5	Dislocated joints.
	Loose joints (moxa more affective).

Kidney

Best formula to strengthen Ki chi
= Bl 23, Ki3, GV4.

Bl 23	Adjusts Ki chi.

CV 4	Builds up the Ki and firms up the body foundation.
CV 6	Tonifies the Ki.
GV 3	Adjusts Ki chi.
GV 4	Tonifies the Ki and Ki yang.
GV26	Kidney problems.
Ki 3	Benefits empty Ki yin. Benefits the Ki.
Ki 7	Adjusts Ki chi and tonifies the Ki.
Sp 6	Strengthens the Ki.

Knee problems

GV 2	Painful knees.
Ki 7	This point controls the knees.
Ki10	Moxa to strengthen weak knees.
St35	Local point for arthritic knees (and Bl 54).
St36	Sports injuries. St36 to reduce swelling. Li3 for muscles. Bl 60 for pain. St35 knee eyes. GB34 for muscular problems. Bl 54. Crane wind. GB31.

Labour

Bl 67	Difficult labour due to improperly positioned foetus.
CV 2	Uterus returning to normal size after birth.
Ki 9	Massage in 3rd and 6th month of pregnancy to increase health of baby and its resistance to disease.
Pe 6	Excessive bleeding after childbirth – with Sp points. Nausea and vomiting in pregnancy.
Sp 4	Stretch marks after pregnancy.
TH 6	Excessive bleeding after childbirth.

Lactation deficiency

CV 8	Stops excessive milk production.
CV17	Insufficient milk.
Ki 9	
Pe 1	

SI 1
St18

Leg problems

Bl 54	Sports injuries – calf muscles. With Bl 57, Bl 60, Sp6, GB34.
Bl 57	Sports injuries. With Sp6, Bl 54, GB34.
Bl 59	Pain in thigh.
GB30	Any problem of hip.
GB31	Arthritis of hip or knee.
GB35	Neuralgia of leg.
GB36	Calf spasm. Weakness and pain in leg.
Ki 9	Weak legs.
Li 6	Leg pain.
Sp 9	Weak legs. Sports injuries. Good for knee and muscle injuries around area.
St40	Leg paralysis.

Liver

Bl 18	Benefits the Li.
Bl 19	Cools clears and disperses evil heat of the GB and Li.
GB34	Benefits the Li.
GB37	Adjusts and cools the Li.
GB40	Soothes and benefits the Li.
GB41	Disperses the Li and GB.
GV20	Calms the Li (excess conditions) and extinguishes Li wind.
Li 2	Disperses the fire in the Li.
Li 3	Balances the Li. Very useful in empty Li yin problems.
Li 4	Regulates the harmonizing effect of the Li. Used particularly for a stuck condition of the Li.
Sp 6	Opens up and softens the Li.
St 2	Assists the Li in its dispersing function.

Lungs

Bl 12	Assists in the circulation of Lu energy (used in the first stage of an external Lu problem).
Bl 13	Adjusts the Lu.
Bl 38	Regulates Lu chi.
Co20	Disperses wind heat in the Lu.
CV22	Assists in the circulation function of the Lu.
GV12	Lu problems.
Lu 1	All lung disorders.
Lu 5	Controls rebellion of chi in the Lu. Disperses heat in the Lu.
Lu 6	Adjusts and sends down Lu energy.
Lu 7	Circulates Lu energy in general.
Lu 9	Regulates the Lu.
Lu10	Clears heat in the Lu.
Lu11	Cools the Lu.

Lymphatic

Ki 9	Moxa to drain lymphatic system.
Pe 7	Lymphatic problems – with Sp points.

Meningitis

Lu11

Menopause

CV 1.5	Menopause problems.
St30	Menopausal problems.

Menstruation

CV 3	Irregular periods.
Ki 4	Painful menstruation and associated emotional problems.
Ki 5	Premenstrual tension.
Li 2	Irregular menses.
Pe 6	Disturbed menses.
Sp 6	Menstruation regulation with Pe6. With Co4 for bringing on period.
Sp 8	Painful menses.
Sp 9	Menstrual problems.

Sp10   Irregular periods.

Meridian stagnation
Bl 1   Moves the meridians.
Co 4   Moves the face meridians.
Co14   Moves the meridians.
Co15   Moves the meridians.
Co16   Moves the meridians.
St 6   Moves the meridians.
St34   Moves the St meridian (therefore indicated for leg problems).
TH 5   Moves the meridians and stuck chi. Moves the yang of the body.
TH 8   Moves and opens up the upper yang meridians. TH8 is the meeting point for yang in the upper part of the body.

Migraine
Bl 10   With GB20 and GB21.
Co 4
CV12   With CV4 for migraine due to premenstrual tension.
CV15
GB20   With GB21 and Bl10.
GB41   Very useful for migraine.
GV24.5
Ht 7
Ki 6   Due to premenstrual syndrome.
St40
TH 3

Mucus
Lu 9   Transforms mucus, and aids in the circulation of damp sputum.
Pe 5   Expels mucus in the chest (Tan yin obstructs the function of the Ht).
Sp 2   Expels mucus caused by weak Sp (i.e., Sp sending up dirty energy to the Lu).
St40   General point for all mucus problems as it transforms mucus.

Mumps
TH17

Muscle – see limb problems etc.
Co 5
Sp11   Sports injuries. Muscular injuries
with Sp10, Sp6, Bl 60 for pain.
St31   Strained thigh muscles – footballers
injuries. St31, St36, St44. Sedate if
heavy drainage of energy. Also use
Co4 as a supplement. GB34. Bl 60
for pain.

Nausea
Bl 54

Neck problems – see shoulder problems
GB21   Sports injuries resulting in stiff neck.
With GB20, TH3 and special point
between 2nd and 3rd metacarpals.

Nervousness
Ht 4   Calm with Ht,4,5,6,7
Pe 6   With TH5 for nervous breakdown.
TH 7   Nervous trembling.

Obesity
Bl 54

Palpitations
Ht 6
Ht 7

Pancreas
Sp 6

Paralysis
Co10   Hemiplegia.
CV23
GV14

GV15
Ht 1   Paralysis of all limbs.
Ki 8   Lower limb paralysis.
Li 6
Lu 5   Hemiplegia.

Parkinson's disease
Co11   Special point for Parkinson's disease
              (or any shaking of extremeties).

Pleurisy
TH 6

Prostate
St29   Prostate and Gonads.

Quadraplegia
Bl 30
Bl 59
Lu 5

Rectum
CV 4   Rectum prolapse with GV1.
GV 1   Rectum prolapse with GV20.
GV20   Rectal prolapse.

Rheumatism
Co10   With St36 to tonify energy in cases
              of rheumatism.

Rheumatoid arthritis
Bl 58

Schizophrenia
GV14

Shock
GV20
GV26
Ki 1   Brings out of shock – will cause to
              cry and urinate.
Ki 5   After slight shock.

Ki 6	Emergency point for concussion and unconsciousness.
Pe 6	
SI 1	
SI 3	Slow recovery from shock.
Sp 1	Good for use after shock.
Sp 3	Eliminates post trauma shock (especially with amnesia) – i.e., after affects of shock due to bad memories.

Shoulder problems

Co15	
	Sports injuries. With Co15, Co16, SI11, Co11.
GV14	Neck tension and shoulder problems.
Lu 2	Local point for shoulder neuralgia.
SI 3	Shoulder pain. Shoulder relaxation. Twisted back on opposite side.
St38	Frozen shoulder – often immediate results.
TH 3	Back and shoulder problems.
TH11	
TH14	

Sinus

Co 4	With Co20
GV24.5	

Skin

Bl 62	Painful skin.
Bl 65	Skin problems. Abscesses.
Co 1	Acne on the face.
Co 4	Skin problems.
Co 5	Increases energy on skin surface.
Co11	Dry skin.
GV14	Skin eruptions.
Sp10	2 up is special skin point (nest of 100 caterpillars) with Co11.
St 5	Facial Acne.

Small intestine

Bl 27	Moves and adjusts the St.
Pe 3	Adjusts the intestines.

Smoking

CV15	Anti smoking.
CV17	Anti smoking point (back up with shenmen and Lu points). Plus ears-shenmen and 2Lu.

Spirit or shen

Bl 15	Pacifies the spirit.
Bl 62	Clears and cools the spirit – has a very strong effect on the spirit, hence good for insomnia epilepsy etc.
Bl 64	Calms the spirit.
CV14	Calms the spirit.
GV20	Pacifies the spirit.
Ht 3	Quietens the shen.
Ht 5	Quietens the shen.
Ht 7	Pacifies the spirit (most important point for the spirit).
Ht 8	Quietens the shen.
Ki 6	Calms the spirit.
Pe 4	Calms the spirit.
Pe 5	Calms the spirit.
Pe 7	Quietens the spirit.

Spleen

Bl 20	Adjusts Sp chi. Helps the transformation and moving aspects of the Sp. Therefore it is good for strengthening and unblocking or ensuring Sp energy is moving in the right direction.
CV 8	Strengthens the transforming power of the Sp. The point of choice in problems of Sp yang weak.
Sp 1	Benefits the Sp.
Sp 2	Tonifies the Sp.
Sp 5	Strengthens Sp yang in general. Strengthens the Sp and St.

Sp 6	Strengthens the Sp.
St36	Regulates the Sp.

Stings

Ki 6	Massage for wasp, gnat and bee stings.

Stomach

Bl 21	Adjusts St chi.
Bl 25	Adjusts the St.
CV 8	Rids excess St gas. Stomach ache.
CV12	Adjusts the St.
CV14	Harmonizes the St.
Pe 5	Harmonizes the St.
Pe 7	Harmonizes the St.
Sp 5	Strengthens the Sp and St.
Sp 6	Gastro intestinal disorders with St36.
St34	Gastralgia. Harmonizes the St in excess conditions.
St36	Regulates the St.
St37·	Regulates the St.
St41	Tonifies the St. Cold damp stomach (indigestion from unripe fruit) – warms the stomach.

Sweating

Co 4	Causes sweating (tonifies Wei Chi).
GB41	Excessive perspiration.
Ht 1	Excessive perspiration with general weakness.
Ht 6	Night sweats with SI3.
Ki 7	With Co4 for excessive sweating without cause – will dry up in minutes.
Pe 9	Induces sweating.
SI 4	Use with Ki7 for excessive sweating.
TH10	Excessive perspiration.

Talking

St40   Stops people continually talking.

Teeth problems – see also facial problems

Co 1   Toothache on opposite side of face.

GV27   Toothache.

St 5   Local point for toothache.

St42

St45   St45-42 for mouth afflictions (e.g., toothache).

Tension

GV 8   Extreme tension – pent up anger.

GV12   Extreme tension.

SI 3

Throat problems

CV22.5   Finger pressure for a few minutes will cure sore throat.

Ki 3   Dry throat. Mouth and throat problems.

Lu 7   Throat infections.

SI 7   Acute throat pain.

St44   Sore throat.

Thyroid

Co 1   Has direct affect on due to lung connection.

Sp 6

Tinnitus

GB 2

Pe 9

SI 2

SI19

TH 2

TH 3

TH17

TH21

Tonsils

Co 4

SI17   With Co4 .

Trigeminal neuralgia
    SI19

Ulcers

	Duodenal ulcers caused by Sp.
	Stomach ulcers caused by Li.
Bl 54	Gastric and duodenal ulcers.
CV12	Local point for ulcers.

Vagus

CV22	Has direct effect on vagus nerve.

Vomiting

CV12	Special point for vomiting.
CV24	Prevents vomiting in females.
St12	Good for nausea and vomiting due to dialysis machine.
	Prevents vomiting (particularly in male).
TH19	Vomiting in children.

Whiplash

GB39	Use on opposite side.

Wind

Bl 1	Expels wind.
Bl 12	Expels wind.
Bl 60	Disperses wind in the head.
Bl 64	Disperses wind.
Co 1	Controls wind caused by heat.
Co 4	Expels wind.
Co11	Expels wind.
GB13	Disperses wind.
GB20	Moves wind. An important point for all wind in the body either internal or external.
Lu 7	Disperses wind.
Lu 9	Disperses wind.
St 2	Expels wind.
St 6	Expels wind.
TH17	Disperses wind.

Yang

Bl 17	Reunion point of yin and yang in the body.
CV 4	Main tonification point for the yang in the body.
CV12	Influential point for the yang organs.
GB39	Connects the 3 lower yang. Group Luo.
GV14	Meeting point of all the yang meridians.
Lu 7	Takes energy out of the lung into the 6 yang. General Luo.
Pe 6	Takes energy from all yin to the yang (this balances yin yang on a large scale). General Luo.
TH 8	Meeting point for yang in the upper part of the body. Moves and opens up the upper yang meridians. Group Luo.

Yin

Bl 17	Reunion point of yin and yang of the body.
CV 6	General source point for lower yin energy.
CV15	General source point for upper yin energy.
Li13	Influential point for yin organs.
Pe 5	Balances upper yin. Group Luo.
Sp 6	Meeting point of 3 lower yin.
TH 5	Takes energy from all the yang to the yin (this balances yin and yang on a large scale). General Luo.

Triple Heater

Bl 26	Regulates the lower heater.
Bl 31	Regulates the lower heater.
Bl 32	Regulates the lower heater.
Bl 33	Regulates the lower heater.
Bl 34	Regulates the lower heater.
TH 4	Moves the meridian.

BIBLIOGRAPHY

Acupuncture. A report to the National Health and Medical Research Council (The Australian Government).

American Journal of Acupuncture from 1973 to 1980.

Austin, M. *Acupuncture Therapy.* Turnstone Press, Wellingborough, Northants., 1974.

A Barefoot Doctors Manual. (The American Translations of the official Chinese paramedical manual). Running Press, Philadelphia, U.S.A. 1977.

Duke, M. *Acupuncture.*

Huard, P. and Wong M. *Chinese Medicine.*

Jayasuriya, A. *Acupuncture Therapeutics.*

Kushi, M. *Oriental Diagnosis.* Sunwheel Publications, London, 1978.

Mann, F. *Acupuncture the Ancient Chinese Art of Healing and How it Works Scientifically.* Heinemann, London, 1978.

Mann, F. *The Meridians of Acupuncture.* Heinemann, London, 1964.

Mann, F. *The Treatment of Disease by Acupuncture.* Heinemann, London, 1974.

Porkert, M. *The Theoretical Foundations of Chinese Medicine.* M.I.T. Press, Cambridge, Massachusetts, U.S.A., 1974.

The Yellow Emperor's Classic of Internal Medicine. (Translated by Ilza Veith)

Various lecturers for Acupuncture Colleges (Australia).

An intensive course in Chinese Medicine conducted by Christopher Madden.

INDEX

abdomen, 25, 26, 54
alcoholics, 37, 44, 47, 48
allergies, 33
ankle, 55
anuria, 42
arthritis, 39

bacteria, 10
back, 54
bladder, 42, 56
body fluids, 12-17, 21, 22, 29, 36, 38, 40, 42, 44, 46, 47, 50, 54
brain, 12
spinal, 12

carbon dioxide, 11
chi, 10-18, 23, 24, 27, 29, 35-37, 39, 40, 41, 45, 47-49, 52-54
chen, 11, 12, 33
ching, 12, 54
ku, 11
tsing, 12
wei, 11
ying, 12
cold, 29-30
colon, 12, 38, 42, 55, 56
spastic, 22
constipation, 22, 41, 42
cough, 15, 31
cyanosis, 15, 38, 48

dampness, 10, 30-31
diabetes, 12, 37, 41
diarrhoea, 22, 31, 42
diet, 10, 15, 26, 40
digestion, 14, 31, 35, 37, 41, 49, 54
diptheria, 39
disease classification, 19
dizziness, 15, 27, 28
dryness, 10, 31
dysentry, 42

ears, 40
edema, 12, 30, 37, 42
elbow, 56
eyes, 12, 34, 36-37
spots in front of, 16, 27

face, 14, 16, 17, 24, 27, 30
black, 35
flushing, 24

green, 36
pallor, 22-23
red, 34
white, 35
yellow, 34-35
faeces, 42
feet, 55
fever, 26, 29, 30
fingernails, 16, 39-40

gall bladder, 41, 51, 55, 56
gums, 38

hands, 56
haemorrhage, 15, 16
nasal, 30
heart, 9, 11, 32, 37, 41, 44, 45, 47
heat fire, 30
hip, 56

incontinence, 15, 42
insomnia, 16, 41
intestine, 14, 16, 42, 50, 51, 52
small, 12, 38, 56

jaundice, 34

kidney, 9, 11, 12, 15, 33, 35-39, 41, 42, 44, 45, 48, 50, 51, 54, 55, 56
knee, 55-56

legs, 56
liver, 9, 12, 32, 36-39, 41, 43-47, 50, 51, 55
lungs, 11, 12, 14, 15, 26, 30, 31, 32, 35, 37, 38, 39

mouth, 37-38
menstruation, 43
meridians, 14, 15, 16, 25, 30, 39
mucus, 12, 16, 22, 23, 35, 38, 41, 49, 50, 51, 52, 54
nasal, 43
muscles, 12, 44, 53

nocturia, 42
nose, 37, 43
bleed, 16, 37

obesity, 34
oliguria, 42

parasites, 35, 37, 41
pathogens, 15, 20
pericardium, 41, 44, 45, 55, 56
photophobia, 36, 37
Pill, the, 35
polyuria, 42
pulse, 14, 15, 16, 18, 23-27, 29-31
diagnosis, 20, 52-56

rectum, 42
respiration, 15, 18, 24, 25, 53

saliva, 12, 21, 38, 50
shen, 33, 41
shoulders, 34
Six Excesses, the, 28
skin, 12, 16, 18, 25, 26, 29, 30, 31, 38, 52
spleen, 9, 11, 14, 28, 32, 35, 37, 38, 40-45, 47, 49-52, 55, 56
sputum, 43
stomach, 9, 12, 14, 26, 35, 37-42, 44, 50, 51, 54-56

Tao, 9
teeth, 38, 44
tendons, 12, 25, 39, 44
throat, 26, 27, 29, 39
tinnitus, 15, 29
tiredness, 14, 27
tongue, 15, 16, 17, 18, 20, 23, 24, 27, 30, 31, 43-52
diagnosis, 20
moss, 49-52

urine, 12, 14, 15, 22, 27, 31, 42

virus, 52
pathogenic, 10
vomiting, 26, 27, 31, 42

wind, 10, 28-29

yin and yang, 9, 10, 14-18, 21, 22, 24, 27-31, 34-42, 44, 47-50, 52, 53, 54
functions of organs, 11-12
illness, 28